HATHA YOGA:

Developing the Body, Mind and Inner Self

2nd Edition

Dee Ann Green Birkel, M.A.
Assistant Professor
Ball State University
Muncie, Indiana

eddie bowers publishing inc.
2600 Jackson Street
Dubuque, Iowa 52001-3342

ACKNOWLEDGEMENTS

I wish to thank many people for their contributions to this second edition. First I wish to thank my family: Mary for the thorough editing of the manuscript; Becky for the section on Acupuncture and Acupressure; my son Jeff and daughter-in-law Tammy for their beautiful children, Katie, Matt and Mike who did "Yoga" for Grandmother's camera; and to my husband Lane, daughter Laura and sons-in-law Tom and Ron for their encouragement and support.

A thank you also to the photographer of the first edition, Paul Troxell and for the second edition Dave Thurston. Also for technical assistance I would like to thank Associate Dean Jean Wittig for her computer support and Brad Slack for the computer drawings. Thanks also to massage therapist/educator, Ruth Ann Hobbs, to chiropractor, Dexter Nardella, and to Trager Practioner, Michael Sternfeld for sharing their knowledge and expertise with me. To my colleagues in the Womens Physical Education Department, The School of Physical Education and at Ball State University who have supported hatha yoga in the curricululm another big THANK YOU!

To all of you great Ball State University Students who volunteered to be the models: Maria Sharp, Kevin Raidy, Gary Telles, Beth Bowser and Jim Enyart who posed for the majority of the asanas; to Shawn Yancy who demonstrated yoga asanas while pregnant; to Tara Maxberry and her guide dog Megan; and to the athletes: Mary Beth Singleton, Gena Rusch, Dave Keener, Steve Alexander, Amy Boras, Julie Focht, Stacy Jones, Daniele Poquette, Ryan Reed, Angie Sunier, and Bonzi Wells thanks for the photos and the good time. I cherish your sharing and the memories of the photo sessions.

And to all of my hatha yoga teachers and my hatha yoga students who have all taught me so much, I wish to express my appreciation and gratitude.

And finally, thanks to Margaret at eddie bowers publishing, inc. for bringing this second edition to its final stage.

NAMASTE,
Dee Ann
Fall, 1995

COVER PHOTO: BALL STATE STUDENTS left to right:
    1st Row: Dee Ann Birkel and Megan, the guide dog.
    2nd. Row: Angie Sunier, Tracy Jones, Tara Maxberry, and Amy Boras
    3rd Row: Dani Poquette, Rachel Beltrane, Beth Bowser, and Julie Focht
    4th Row: Steve Alexander, Bonzi Wells, Ryan Reed, and Jim Enyart

eddie bowers publishing, inc.
2600 Jackson Street
Dubuque, Iowa 52001-3342

ISBN 0-945483-59-7

TABLE OF CONTENTS

Preface v

Unit 1 Introduction: What is Yoga? 1
Yoga in the United States 1
International Yoga Scene 2
Potential for Self Growth 3
Summary 4
Resources 4

Unit 2 Yoga Basics 7
Self Assessment 7
Body Composition and Flexibility 7
Resting Pulse 8
Weight 8
Height 8
Girth Measurements 8
Hip to Waist Ratio 9
Flexibility 9
Sit and Reach 9
Hip Flexibility 9
Shoulder Flexibility 10
Trunk Lift 10
Hatha Yoga Practice Guidelines 11
Attitudinal 11
Practical 11
Summary 12
Resources 12

Unit 3 Asanas: Hatha Yoga Poses 13
The "ABC'S" of Hatha Yoga 13
Awareness & Concentration 13
Breath 13
Counterpose 13
Preparation Poses 14
Neck Stretch 14
Neck Turn 14
Body Rolls 14
Knee Thigh Stretch 15
One Knee to Chest 15
Diagonal Knee to Chest 15
Shoulder & Back Stretch at Wall
or Ballet Barre 16
Thigh Toner 16
Head Lift & Turn 16
Feldenkrais Kneeovers 17
Toe-Hold Leg Lift 17
Alternate Leg Stretch 18
Asanas 19
Mountain Pose 19
Cobra 20
Cobra with Head Turn 20
Half Locust 21
Fetus 22
Knees to Chest 22
Sitting Forward Bend 23
Head of Cow 24
Chest Expansion 25
Cat 26
Cat "Push-Up and Down" 27
Dog 28
Yoga Sit Back & UP 29
Shoulderstand 30
Fish 33
Spinal Twist 34

Tree 35
Triangle 36
Triangle Twist 37
Abdominal Lift 38
Back Push-Up 39
Lion 40
Dolphin 41
Moon Salute Routine 42
Beginning Yoga Practice Session 43
Summary 44
Resources 44

Unit 4. Asanas: Intermediate Hatha Yoga
Poses 45
Lunge 45
Plank 46
Flying Locust 46
Full Locust 47
Headstand Hang 48
Headstand 49
Arrow Sit 50
Rishi 50
Balance Posture 51
Camel 51
Bow 52
Half Boat 52
Standing Straddle Forward Bend . 53
Warrior I 54
Warrior II 55
Warrior III 56
Half Moon 57
Half Lotus & Lotus 58
Plough 59
Routines or "Postural Flows" 60
Crocodile Routine 60
Salute to the Sun 61
Vinyasa 62
Partner Yoga 63
Ashtanga Vinyasa Yoga -
(Power Yoga) 67
22 Step Variation of Sun Salute 68
Power Yoga Routine 70
Intermediate Level Teachers 70
Iyengar Classes 70
Ganga White and Tracy Rich 70
Kalli Ray 70
Resources 71

Unit 5 Pranayama: Breathing Techniques 73
What is Pranayama 73
Benefits 73
Recommendations 74
Varieties of Yoga Breathing 75
Complete Breath with *UJJAYI* 75
Ha Breath with Abdominal Lift 75
Alternate Nostril Breath 76
Yoga Nasal Cleansing Process:
NETI 77
Kapalabhati 78
Bellows Breath 78
Yoga Breathing for Asthmatics and
Other Lung Conditions 78
Summary 79
Resources 79

iv

PREFACE

This book has grown from the need to have an appropriate Hatha Yoga text book for college classes. I have been teaching in the University setting since 1977. This book is directed toward the beginning student with material presented in a format that is easily understood and used in a practice session. Many of the ideas and content in this book are the result of a survey given to my students. They were asked to tell me what THEY wanted in a book and what THEY thought would be helpful to them.

Yoga is no longer regarded by our society as an activity that is mysterious. Thousands are learning and practicing yoga in their own living room via a videotape or a television program. Some become acquainted with yoga at health/fitness spas and many have taken yoga at YMCA's and YWCA's, open universities, weekend workshops and on college campuses. Yoga has become an accepted form for helping with stress reduction as well as having a teaching format that is non-competitive and individualized.

Yoga has been recommended by physicians, psychologists, psychiatrists, chiropractors, massage therapists and athletic trainers to people of all sizes, shapes and ages. This second edition includes in Unit 9, further discussion of yoga's therapeutic application in our society. We have become even more aware of our "whole self" and that we do not just consist of unrelated parts. We are interconnected and the learning of yoga assists in this discovery so that our marvelous machine, the human body and inner self, can reach its full potential.

This book will discuss the yoga exercises and how they help the body develop muscle strength, endurance, flexibility, balance, breath control and mental concentration. This second edition includes more challenging asanas in Unit 4. Let me stress that everyone is different and we come in all forms. Each of us is an unique individual and thus the approach to hatha yoga is one that encourages each person to work at a level that is comfortable.

This book includes check sheets as well as a list of references for supplemental reading. This book provides, for college and high school students in particular, and any other beginning student of yoga, a practical introductory guide to hatha yoga.

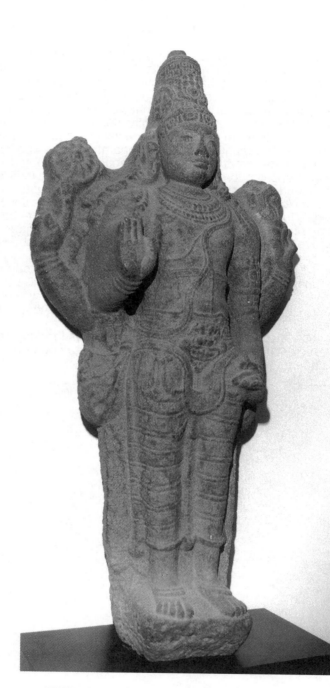

VISHNU, Indian, Chola period 1100-1399
Unidentified maker, stone

Photo loaned by Ball State University Museum of Art, Muncie, IN., lent by David T. Owsley 191.042.8

The ancient cultures of the world, the Greeks, Romans, Celts, have often depicted their deities and mythological figures in art work. This is also true of India where the above figure was carved. Standing in a squarely frontal position, this figure of the Hindu deity Vishnu is the picture of reserved emotion. With a knowing smile on his full mouth and his eyes wide open, Vishnu stands with his primary right hand in the *abhaya mudra*, the left relaxed on his upper thigh; his secondary hands hold two of his attributes, the *padma* and *sankha*.

As one of the three deities of the Hindu trinity, or *Trimurti*, Vishnu intends only good. Wearing a jewel on his breast and a diadem on his head, Vishnu holds his attributes of the discus, shell, club and lotus in his four arms. Often shown seated on his mighty stead, the great eagle Garuda, he is a god of kindness and benevolence.

Introduction: What is Yoga

> *When we treat Man as he is,*
> *we make him worse than he is.*
> *When we treat him as if he already were*
> *what he potentially could be,*
> *we make him what he should be.*
> **Goethe (1749-1832)**

YOGA can be defined as a "way of life" which developed in India approximately 5,000 years ago. It is a system of working with the whole body. The word "YOGA" is derived from the Sanskrit word "yuj" from which we get the word yoke or union, meaning to join or unite together all aspects of us as a person-our physical self, our mental self, our emotional self, our history, and our goals for the future. We are not just a body that is strengthening muscles, improving range of motion at the joints, practicing a stress reduction technique such as relaxing, or improving energy and lung capacity by doing the breathing techniques. These are all important components but when they are all incorporated into one Hatha Yoga exercise session the effect on the body and the benefits gained are marvelous to experience. I have heard so many wonderful stories from my 6000 -plus students since 1977 of how the class has helped them cope, improve some aspect of their life or even changed their lives in some way for the better.

HATHA YOGA is one aspect of the multifaceted nature of yoga. The main stages of yoga are known as:

Jnana Yoga - Union by developing knowledge

Bhakti Yoga - Union by developing love and devotion

Karma Yoga - Union by practicing service and being active

Mantra Yoga - Union by using the voice and sound

Kundalina Yoga - Union by developing the chakra system

Hatha Yoga - Union by developing the body and breath

Raja Yoga - Union by mastering mental capacity

In the practice of hatha yoga the concentration is on the physical exercises (the asanas), and the breathing techniques (the pranayama), and the learning of relaxation techniques. The word "HATHA" is really two words from Sanskrit -"HA" means Sun and "THA" means Moon. This implies that as the forces from the Sun and Moon interact upon us and keep us and our universe in balance, we are to strive for this same balance in ourselves as well.

The history of yoga is long and interesting. It is believed to have developed in Northern India about 5,000 years ago as a means of training soldiers. It wasn't until the 5th or 6th century B.C. that scholars say that an Indian philosopher, Pantanjali, formulated the early yoga teachings into a science of physical and mental health that are known today as the *"Yoga Sutras."*

Yoga in the United States

Yoga has been of interest to many Americans for over 200 years. In 1794, Thomas Jefferson read the recent translation by Sir William Jones of *The Institutes of Hindu Law: or the Ordinances of Manu.* In 1805 William Emerson, father of Ralph Waldo Emerson was the editor of the magazine, *The Monthly Anthology and Boston Review,* which published the first English translation of the Sanskrit manuscript, *Sacontala.*

In 1842, Emerson and Thoreau published translations of Hindu scriptures. In 1843, in Concord, Massachusetts, three famous Americans, Ralph Waldo Emerson, Henry David Thoreau and Bronson Alcott undertook an intellectual study of the ancient writings of India from the book known as the *Bhagavad Gita".* It was in 1893 that the first Indian teacher, Swami Vivekananda, came to the United States, arriving in Chicago to give a speech to the World Parliament of Religions. He stayed for two years giving lectures in Detroit, Boston, New York and Chicago. In 1899 he founded the New York Vedanta

Society and four of his colleagues opened yoga centers (known as ashrams) near Los Angeles and in San Francisco. The interest in yoga continued to grow with the arrival of more teachers from India :

1920 - Paramahansa Yogananda in Boston
1922 - Jiddu Krishnamurti and his brother Nitya to Ojai, CA
1927 - L. Adams Beck published *A Beginner's Book of Yoga*
1947 - Indra Devi, first woman teacher and student of Sri Krishnamacharya opened a yoga studio in Hollywood
1953 - Indra Devi publishes *Forever Young, Forever Healthy.*
1961 - Swami Vishnudevanada, started the Sivananda Yoga Centers, in Val Morin, Quebec, Montreal, New York City, and at Nassau in the Bahamas
1961 - Richard Hittlelman started the first nationally televised hatha yoga program
1964 - Marcia Moore opened a yoga studio at Concord, MA and became the subject of the popular book *Yoga, Youth and Reincarnation,* by Jess Stearns
1968 - Swami Kriyananda founded a residential community near Nevada City, CA
1966 - Swami Satchidananda became known as the "Guru of Woodstock"

There were more students of Sri Krishnmacharya who continued to make a tremenduous impact on the American Hatha yoga scene and who are still active-

1973 - B.K.S. Iyengar
1975 - Pattabhi Jois
1976 - T.K.V. Desikachar (son of Krishnamacharya)
1970 - Lilias Folan launched the first PBS-TV series "Lilias, Yoga & You", which by 1977 was broadcast over 200 stations
1970 - Swami Rama of the Himalayan Institute was involved in the research conducted at the prestigious Menninger Foundation in Topeka, KA where he demonstrated yogic control over involuntary autonomic nervous system function, including heartbeat, pulse rate and skin temperature, which contributed to the development and growth of the science of biofeedback
1970 - Norman Allen became the first American to accomplish the full ashtanga yoga series of Pattabhi Jois (later known as "power yoga")
1971 - Swami Rama established the Himalalyan International Institute of Yoga Science and Philosophy in Chicago, IL
1973 - B.K.S. Iyengar came to Ann Arbor, MI. Also, the first retreat center, the 3HO,

was established in Tucson AZ, using yoga to treat addictions
1974 - In San Francisco, Rama Vernon and Rose Garfinkle published a newsletter *The Word*, which was the parent of the *Yoga Journal*
1977 - Ball State University, School of Physical Education, Muncie, IN offered hatha yoga classes for college credit

Yoga has thus become assimiliated into our American culture and is currently not being presented in a rigid, religious, style but more as a philosophy or a way of life. According to results of a Roper poll reported in an article in *Mens Health* , (May 1995 p. 86)-"traditional yoga has a fairly strong U.S. following - 6 million." There are also highly visible USA citizens, actors, actresses, athletes, politicians, etc., who practice yoga and share with others their involvement via articles, interviews, and video tapes.

Following is a partial list for your information.

Sting - musician
Kareen Abdul-Jabbar - basketball player
Shirley Mcclain - actress
Warren Beatty - actor
Racquel Welch - actress
Ali Mc Graw - actress
Olivia Newton-John - singer
Jack Niklaus - golfer
Gail Sheehy - author
Ringo Starr - musician
Dolly Parton - singer
Jackie Kennedy Onassis (deceased)

International Yoga Scene

Yoga, like music, art, and sports, transcends the globe. One of the most exciting aspects of learning yoga is that no matter where you are in the world you will probably be able to find a class or a friend who also practices yoga. There are many yoga centers throughout the Western World of Europe, England, North and South America as well as in the desirable resort areas of the islands in the Mediteranean, Pacific, Gulf of Mexico and the Atlantic ocean. Many of the leading teachers of one country will travel and do workshops around the world. The masters of yoga from India are well known among the yoga teachers of the world. In this book you will learn of the teachers Swami Dev Murti who lived in England and is now back in India; Mr Iyengar whose book, *Light on Yoga,* is probably the most widely used book in the world, and Ashtanga Yoga or "power yoga" of Pattabhi Jois, which is the style of hatha yoga gaining in popularity in the 1990s.

There is also an international yoga organization, "Unity in Yoga," which sponsors a conference every two years. They , along with the *Yoga Journal,* and Rama Vernon of the Center for Soviet-American Dialogue sponsored a two week yoga conference in Moscow during October of 1990. I attended along with thirty-one "Citizen Diplomats" from all over the United States with a variety of yoga teaching approaches. What we had in common was the desire to become better acquainted with the 300 Soviet conference attendees and to share the common bond of yoga. The ban forbidding Yoga to be taught in the Soviet Union had only been lifted in the past 2-3 years. From the time of the 1917 Revolution yoga had been banned, but some had gone underground to continue their practice. Yoga had a regrowth in the Gorbachev years but as recently as 1986 one of the men attending the conference had spent three years in prison for teaching yoga. There was a strong grass-roots support for this conference and free classes were held in schools all over Moscow. Hundreds waited for several hours for the opportunity to take a class with us (Fig. 1.1). All of us, both Soviet and American, found this to be a very enlightening two weeks. I returned to the United States valuing our right to make decisions for ourselves in regards to our own growth and potential, and not having a government tell us what we can and can not do. These international experiences through yoga greatly enrich one's life.

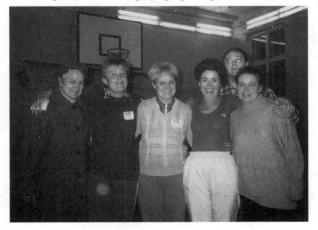

Figure 1.1   *1990 Russian American Yoga Conference*

To become informed on the possibilities available for you to pursue an international yoga experience refer to the *Yoga Journal* for the annual directory of yoga retreats, camps, trips, teacher training centers and teachers throughout the world (refer to resources).

Potential for Self Growth

I would like to share with you the results of a research project conducted at Ball State University by Susan Gove Rudolph for her doctoral dissertation in 1981. The intent of the project was to determine if those 54 female students who participated in the ten week Hatha Yoga class could produce a change in self-concept. The results were compared with the 53 female students in an Effective Interpersonal Relationship Development class taught by Counselling Psychology and 53 female students in four randomly selected algebra classes. All of the subjects were given a questionnaire (Bills Index of Adjustment and Values) at the beginning and end of the ten week sessions. The students in the Hatha Yoga group indicated a significant change in self-concept (p=.006) but not the Counseling Psychology group (p =.08) or the comparison group of Algebra students (p=.36). As these young women participated in the Hatha Yoga class, the discrepancy between how they saw themselves and how they would like to be, decreased. "The majority of the students who answered a Student Opinion Questionnaire felt that participation in the Hatha Yoga class had helped them become more aware of themselves, feel better about themselves and had helped them solve personal and/or physical problems"(Rudolph, Abstract p. 4, resources). I was very excited about these findings as we now had proof of a scientific nature of the far reaching and positive effects of doing Hatha Yoga. Students at this stage in their life are very vulnerable and under pressure from society to be a certain way in regards to body build, looks, clothes, etc., and thus can feel dissatisfied with themselve quite easily. Through the participation in the yoga activity, which was essentially the same that term as every other term before and since, we can conclude that young women can become more accepting of themselves, thus hopefully alleviating some unhappiness and stress in their lives. This finding demonstrates an important contribution on the part of yoga to the overall lifestyle of an individual.

The benefits gained from doing yoga are many and varied depending on the individual's needs. But in general it is safe to say that the basic flexibility, muscular strength, and endurance of the person doing yoga will be enhanced. Also, the awareness of the breath and how the body can control and use the breath for raising energy levels and to calm the self is discovered. One of yoga's main contributions toward self growth is the awareness of the value of relaxation and ways to still the body and the mind . Many students develop a greater awareness of the marvelous ways in which the body is interconnected and how the mind can work with the physical self in a more harmonious manner. Once the practice is established and the attitude toward the self is one of respect, the student then becomes more aware of other lifestyle practices such as good nutrition, and not polluting the body. You will discover that the style and approach of how yoga is done can be transferred to other exercise practices as well.

SUMMARY

Yoga is like any activity you undertake- you get out of it what you put in. What you bring to it in the way of interest and awareness will enhance what you then will see as benefits. Read on now for some basic suggestions on how best to develop and continue your interest in hatha yoga.

We have come to this world to accept it, not merely to know it. We may become powerful by knowledge, but we attain fullness by sympathy. The highest education is that which does not merely give us information, but makes our life grow, in harmony with all existence.

. . . Rabindranath Tagore, 1901.

(recipient of 1913 Nobel Prize for Literature.)

RESOURCES

Books

Boyd, Doug. *Rolling Thunder.* New York, N.Y. : Dell Publishing Co. Inc. 1974.

_____ *Swami: Encounters with Modern Mystics.* Honesdale, PA.: The Himalayan International Institute of Yoga Science and Philosophy of the U.S.A. 1995.

Carr, Rachael. *Be a Frog, A Bird or A Tree.* Garden City, N.Y.: Doubleday and Co. Inc. 1973.

Kiss, Micchaeline. *Yoga for Young People.* Indianapolis, IN.: Bobbs Merrill Co. Inc. 1971.

Lidell, Lucy. *The Sivananda Companion to Yoga.* New York, N.Y.: Simon & Schuster. 1983.

Winding, Eleanor. *Yoga for Musicians and Other Special People.* Sherman Oaks, CA.: Alfred Publishing Co., Inc. 1982.

Publications

American Health: Fitness of Body and Mind, 28 West 23rd Street, New York, N.Y. 10010.

New Realities: Oneness of Self, Mind and Body. 4000 Albemarle St., NW, Washington, DC 20016.

New Age Journal, P. O. Box 53275, Boulder, CO 80321-3275.

Yoga Journal, 2054 University Ave. Berkely, Ca 94794-9975.

Articles

Bera, T.K, et al. "Body composition, cardiovascular endurance and anaerobic power of yogic practioner. " *Indian Journal of Physiology and Pharmacology.* July, 1993. vol. 37 p. 225-8.

Gaudoin, T. "Yoga," *Harpers Bazaar.* October, 1992. p. 205-8.

Gunnell, Ellise. "A Yen for Yoga," USAir Magazine, March 1992. p. 86-90.

Kunes, Ellen. "No Sweat Fitnes," *Working Woman,* April 1990. p.119-20.

Leviton, Richard. "Celebrating 100 Years of Yoga in America," *Yoga Journal,* May/June 1993. p. 67-71.

Stanton, D. "Yoga with Sting at The Ritz." *Esquire.* March, 1993. p. 152-6.

Dissertations

Collins, Lorrie Ann. *Stress Management and Yoga.* Doctoral Thesis, Indiana University, 1982.

Rudolph, Susan Gove. *The Effect on the Self Concept of Participation in Effective Interpersonal Relationships Development Classes.* Doctoral Thesis, Ball State University, Muncie, IN. 1981.

Organizations

Iyengar Yoga Institute of San Francisco. 2404 27th Avenue, San Francisco, CA 94116.

Sivanada Ashram Yoga Retreat, Box N7550, Paradise Island, Nassau, Bahamas (809)326-2402.

Unity in Yoga International, Nancy Ford-Kohne, Executive Director, Yoga and Health Studies Center, 7918 Bolling Dr., Alexandria, VA 22308.

Himalayan Institute, RR 1 Box 400, Honesdale, PA 18431. 1-800-822-4547.

Look well to this day
    for it is life
        the very best of life
in its brief course lie all
the realities and truths of existence
        the joy of growth,
            the splendour of action,
            the glory of power,

For yesterday is but a memory
        and tomorrow is only a vision
            but today if well-lived, makes
every yesterday a memory of happiness
and every tomorrow a vision of hope
        look well therefore to this day.

                    Ancient Sanskrit Poem

Baby Yoga

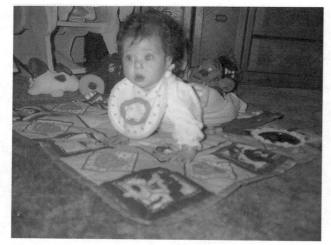

Figure 2.1   *Katie - Cobra at 3 months*

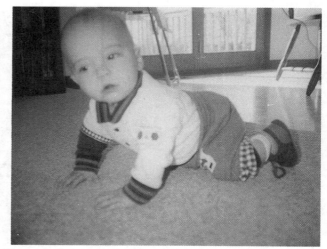

Figure 2.4   *Mike - Cat at 6 months*

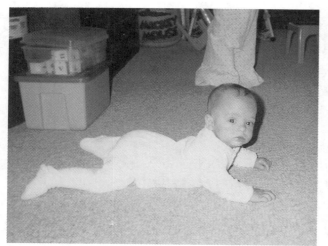

Figure 2.2   *Mike - Cobra with head turn at 5 months*

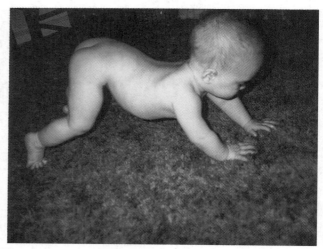

Figure 2.5   *Mike - Dog at 6 months*

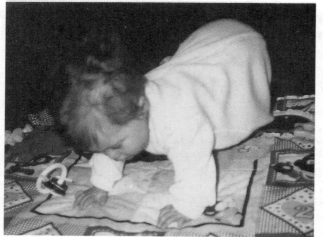

Figure 2.3   *Katie - Dog at 4 months*

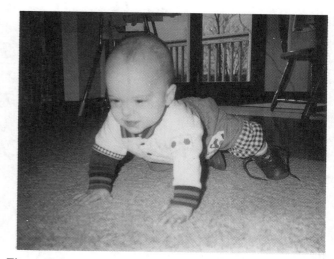

Figure 2.6   *Mike - Plank at 6 months*

YOGA BASICS

> *Don't believe what your eyes are telling.*
> *All they show is limitation.*
> *Look with your understanding,*
> *find out what you already know...*
> . . . Richard Bach, <u>Jonathan Livingston Seagull</u>

The basics of hatha yoga's movement patterns are not new or unusual for our bodies to experience. When I became a grandmother, with appreciation of the wonder of life for these precious little humans, I was enthralled to watch first Katie, then Matt and Mike do "yoga." The very first movement that an infant does is to lift its head and eventually the chest into an "asana" (the Sanskrit word for a yoga pose) known as the COBRA. When the arms are stronger and the co-ordination and motor messages are being established the next asana is the CAT and shortly after that the DOG. When the little body is stronger they begin doing the PLANK. See the accompanying photos of these "Baby Yoga" poses (Fig. 2.1-6). This was a revelation to me - and I have wondered ever since if the ancient founders of yoga developed the asanas with this in mind. So, as a new student of Hatha Yoga, you are really returning to practice the very first movement patterns your neuro-muscular system developed.

SELF ASSESSMENT

To be able to attain as much as possible from your involvement with hatha yoga it is helpful to take a reflective look at your self- your whole self. Ask your self these questions. Who are YOU? What are your hopes and aspirations? What do you really care about? What is your lifestyle like in regard to healthful living? Do you drink, eat, work, or smoke to excess? What are your eating habits? How do you handle stress? Do you exercise now, in the past, or have plans for the present and the future? Do you have any chronic health concerns such as epilepsy, diabetes, migraine headaches, old injuries, pre-menstrual tension, etc.? How do you manage your time? Are your relationships with parents, siblings, roommates, friends, special friends what you want them to be? What are your strengths? What brings you satisfaction? What do you LIKE about yourself?

It is also helpful to complete the Health History Questionnaire, and the Stress Releases and Safety Valves, (Appendices A and C). Refer to unit 6 for more information if your stress score indicates that you are prone to stress problems.

Take a few moments now and write a letter to yourself discussing what ever you think would benefit YOU. You can use the above suggestions but feel free to expand and include anything you want. Now that you have communicated to the very important YOU, why not set a few goals for yourself based upon what developed in your letter ? Be realistic- and don't set too many or set ones that are unattainable at this point in your life. Later, in a few weeks, re-read your letter and at the end of this term or fifteen weeks write yourself another letter relating to the content of your first one. Are there changes in you and how you see who YOU are now? Ask yourself the question— Did yoga play a role in this? The importance of this exercise is to help you become more aware of your whole self, your potential and to appreciate who you are.

BODY COMPOSITION AND FLEXIBILITY

It is also meaningful to assess your physical self. This can be done by following the directions for doing the height, weight, girth measurements, hip to waist ratio, and the flexibility tests and recording them on the Body Analysis Record Form, Appendix B. You will see that there are three columns for recording your data beginning with now, after seven weeks of yoga, and again at the end of fifteen weeks of yoga. Doing it in this manner will allow you to see the changes that are developing.

Resting Pulse

Sit quietly for ten minutes. Find your pulse in your neck or on your wrist and count for 30 seconds and then multiply the number by two thereby giving yourself a pulse count for one minute. A pulse in the range of the sixties or low seventies is considered to be normal. The lower the pulse the less your heart is working at rest. If you have had caffeine or are under stress your pulse could be elevated. A good time to take the pulse for a more accurate count is in the morning just before you get out of bed. As you further your yoga practice and develop your ability to relax, your resting pulse should lower. Take your pulse sometime at the end of your yoga class and see how the relaxation has affected your resting pulse.

Weight

Weigh yourself in your bare or stocking feet, and light weight clothes or in your underwear if possible. Record to nearest 1/4 pound.

Height

Do in your bare or stocking feet, stand erect and have a friend record your height to the nearest 1/4 inch.

Girth Measurements

Refer to the sketch of the body (Fig.2.7) for the location of each site to be measured.

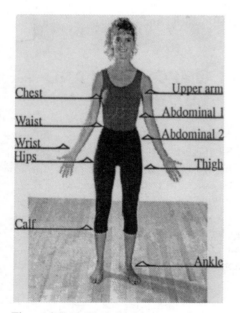

Figure 2.7   *Girth Measurements*

Follow these directions and record your circumference to the nearest 1/4 inch. Please keep the tape level. Measure your right arm and right leg and overlap the tape to get an accurate reading.

Chest: Place the tape over the nipples of the chest and have a friend read the tape in the middle of the back, this allows you to adjust the tape to keep it level.

Abdominal 1: Place the tape just over the bottom of the rib cage.

Waist: Place the tape at the narrowest site for women and for men where you wear your belt.

Abdominal 2: Place the tape over the top of the hip bone (iliac crest on the pelvis).

Hips: Place the tape low over the pubic bone.

Thigh: Near the crotch and keep the tape level!

Calf: Place the tape over the fullest part- where the leg curves.

Ankle: Place the tape just above the bone.

Upper arm: Place the tape near the armpit and keep level!

Wrist: Place the tape just below the bone- toward the hand.

In Table 2.1 you can refer to some Recommended Girth Measurements for Men and Women. These are just a reference if you should want one. No one is expected to be exactly as this would suggest.

Area	Women	Men
Chest	same as hips	same as hips
Abdominal 1		
Waist	10" less than chest	5-7" less than chest
Abdominal 2		
Hips	same as chest	same as chest
Thigh	6" less than waist	8-10 " less than waist
Calf	6-7" less than thigh	7-8" less than thigh
Ankle	5-6" less than calf	6-7" less than calf
Upper arm	twice the size of wrist	twice the size of wrist

Table 2.1   *Recommended Girth Measurements*

Hip to Waist Ratio

The ratio between the measurement of the hip and the waist has been indentified as a method of determining your risk for heart disease. The "apple" shape, when the extra body fat is centered in the chest and abdomen, is at higher risk for high cholsterol, hypertension, and diabetes than the "pear" shape, where the extra body fat is stored on the hips and thighs. The types of fat are different at the two sites. The fat deposited on the hips and thighs is more stagnant and is more difficult to lose. The abdominal fat has more active enzymes and releases more fatty acids into the bloodstream where they can cause trouble. The ratio is computed by dividing the waist measurement by the hip measurement. A ratio for women that is .8 or higher indicates they are at risk and a man with a ratio at .95 or higher is at risk.

Flexibility
Sit and Reach

This test will measure the flexibility of your back and your hamstring muscles on the back of the thigh. To check your flexibility in these areas you will need a "flex-box " (Fig. 2.8), or a chair, a footstool, or a bench laid on its side, as well as a yardstick placed on the edge of the chair with the number 10 on the yardstick lined up with the edge of the chair seat.

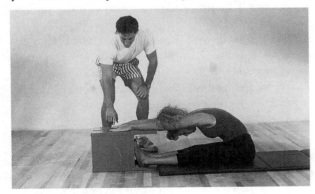

Figure 2.8   *Sit and Reach*

Please follow these instructions.
1. Do a few stretching exercises to gently warm up the muscle groups of the back and legs (See Unit 3 preparation poses).
2. Remove shoes and wear loose clothing.
3. Sit on the floor placing the soles of your feet against the flex box or the chair seat, keeping your legs straight.
4. Place fingertips on your shoulders, INHALE and reach toward the ceiling, straightening arms, lifting ribs, and contracting the abdominal muscles. Then EXHALE and lean for-

ward from the pelvis as far as you can comfortably reach WITHOUT bending your knees. Read the number on the measuring stick where your fingertips touched. If it is beyond the number 10, subtract 10 from the number and write down + _____. If you touched a number from 1 to 10, subtract your number from 10 and write down -_____.

5. Refer to Table 2.2 to see the norms for your reach in inches.

	Men	Women
Excellent	>7.0	>8.5
Good	4.0-7.0	6.5-8.5
Average	1.0-3.9	4.0-6.4
Poor	-2.0-0.9	1.0-3.9
Very Poor	<-2.0	<1.0

From Gwen Robbins, et al., *A Wellness Way of Life,* 2nd edition, Copyright (c) 1994 Wm. C. Brown Communications, Inc. Reprinted with permission of Times Mirror Higher Education Group, Inc., Dubuque, Iowa. All Rights Reserved

Table 2.2

Hip Flexibility

This flexibility test will indicate how flexibile your hip flexors (iliopsoas) are. It is similar to the preparation pose "one knee to chest." Follow these directions.

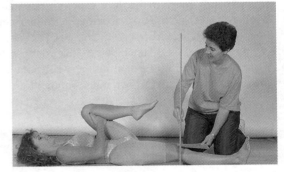
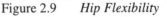

Figure 2.9   *Hip Flexibility*

1. Using a partner to do the measurement, one person lies on their back with the hands on the thigh of **left** leg behind the knee bringing this bent knee to the chest.
2. The other leg is extended straight and if the **right** calf and heel are touching the floor - you record NORMAL.
3. If the **right** calf and heel do NOT touch then the other partner places the yardstick vertical by the outside of the knee and records the number of inches the top of the knee is from the floor.
4. Reverse the leg positions and repeat measuring the **left** leg.

Shoulder Flexibility

This flexibility test will indicate the flexibility of your shoulder girdle. Please follow these directions.

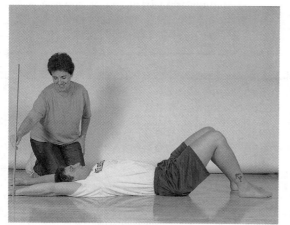

Fig. 2.10   *Shoulder Flexibility*

1. Using a partner to do the measurement, one person lies on their back with both knees bent and your feet flat on the floor.
2. Press down the lumbar area of your back and hold it there with your abdominal muscles as you raise both arms bringing them to rest on the floor behind you.
3. If your hands touch to the floor while you are maintaining contact with the floor with the lumbar area, you record NORMAL.
4. If your hands do NOT touch to the floor your partner places the yardstick vertical by the wrist bone and measures how far EACH wrist is from the floor.

You are never given a wish without also being given the power to make it true.
You may have to work for it however.
. . . Richard Bach, Illusions

Trunk Lift

This flexibility test is similar to a yoga pose that you will be learning. If you have injured your back please don't do it now. If you chose to do it please follow the instructions.

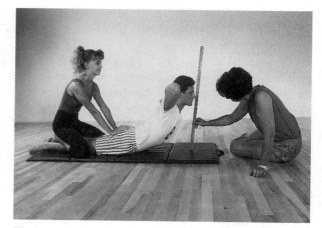

Fig 2.11   *Trunk Lift*

1. Using three partners, one person lies on their abdomen with the fingers interlocked and hands behind the neck. One partner straddles the legs and places his/her hands with the fingers pointing toward the floor on the buttocks and the tops of their feet on the partners ankles to hold the legs down.   The third partner is by the head of the person doing the lift (see Fig. 2.11).
2. The partner on the bottom will inhale and LIFT their trunk upward.   The third partner will place a measuring stick in front of their chin and will quickly record the number of inches (or centimeters) the chin is from the floor.
3. The partner doing the lift will exhale and LOWER down with control.

Hints: Do NOT jerk up quickly and force the body. This should be a gentle lift using the breath and done with control.

Do NOT do this test if you have ever injured the lumbar back or have a problem with the sciatic nerve.

HATHA YOGA PRACTICE GUIDELINES

Please read the following suggestions for participating in a safe and fun hatha yoga session. Most of these recommendations apply to all forms of exercising and are good exercise habits to establish.

The following tips will help you prepare yourself and your attitude toward your yoga practice.

Attitudinal

1. Be constant and serious about your commitment to your practice

2. Set aside a regular time daily - at least 30 minutes

3. Stay focused on what you are doing in that moment and the mind will become quiet

4. Be patient with yourself- don't rush your progress

5. Be an observer - "you" are watching YOU

6. Seek out a state of STILLNESS

7. Let the practice be open and creative- coming from the heart

Practical

1. Begin your practice by focusing on your deep breathing

2. Do the yoga poses 1 1/2 to 2 hours following eating

3. Empty the bladder and bowels

4. Don't chew gum

5. Don't wear large earrings or a lot of jewelry

6. Clothing should be comfortable and allow for movement - NO JEANS! Sweat shirts and pants may be too warm. They also don't allow you to monitor your alignment in the yoga poses

7. Be in bare feet for all of the standing poses. You will have better contact and feedback regarding balance

8. Practice in a well ventilated room and avoid being in a draft

9. Breathe through the nose with the mouth closed. INHALE on the expanding movements and EXHALE on contracting movements. Breathe normally during the static stretching phase

10. Do 3-4 repetitions of each asana

11. If possible check your asanas in a mirror to correct your alignment

12. Don't strain - go to the "edge" of your stretch and back off slightly

13. Concentrate on how your body is feeling and reacting to the activity -involve your mind so that you are more aware of your progress

14. Practice in the early morning is fine but the body is a little stiffer then so be patient and warm up with gentle stretches

15. Evening practice is good as it helps remove the tension of the day and refreshes the mind and body contributing to a sound sleep

16. Always end your practice time with relaxation- you deserve it

17. PRACTICE the basics and MASTER the basics

SUMMARY

Now that you have discovered some very important information about yourself and have learned some guidelines on how to practice, you are ready for the next step: to begin learning the yoga poses and breathing techniques and how they can benefit you. Units 3, 4 and 5 will present this information - so read on.

RESOURCES

Articles

"Yoga Goes Mainstream", *U.S. News and World Report,* May 10, 1994. p. 79-83.

Ingber, D. "Yoga, the Impossible Science," *Science Digest,* February, 1982. p. 28-9.

Lazer, Hart. "Developing Your Own Yoga Practice," *Yoga Journal,* Sept/Oct 1991. p 72,74,115-116.

Stamford, Bryant. "Apples and Pears: Where you 'Wear' Your Fat Can Affect Your Health." *The Physician and Sportsmedicine* 19 (Jan 1991) p 123-24.

Starre, Barbara A. RN, BSN. "Yoga: Progressing Toward High Level Wellness," *Health Valueas* Vol. 13 No.3 May/June 1989, p48-52.

ASANAS: Hatha Yoga Poses

I hear and I forget
I see and I remember
I DO and I understand
. . . A Chinese Proverb

This chapter will introduce you to the yoga poses or "asanas." These exercises are gentle to your body if <u>YOU</u> do them gently. Always move into the pose with control and, as a beginner, you will hold the static stretch or position for approximately ten seconds, then with control, returning to your starting position. Later you will hold in the poses longer. When doing the asanas you are in control of your movements with your mind and breath from the beginning until you send the mental message to complete the pose always ending with control. You are encouraged to refer to the appendix for charts of the muscles and bones, to familiarize yourself with the names as they will be used in the directions and discussions of the yoga asanas.

THE "ABC'S" OF HATHA YOGA

Awareness & Concentration

A concept that is an integral part of yoga practice is "awareness or concentration" - to have your mind FEELING what the physical body is experiencing. Feel the energy needed to do the asana and then feel the relaxation flow through you when you release the contraction or come out of the pose. This feedback can only happen when you have your mind involved and go inward to monitor yourself. **Listen** with your ears to the instructions and also **listen** internally for the body's response. **Think** with your brain about what the body is experiencing and also **think** with the body. Think about how your body is moving internally not only the external view you have if using a mirror. Give the body mental suggestions to "invite" an opening, a releasing, a stretching or a pivoting motion to happen. Incorporating this aware-

ness in to your yoga class and practice from the first day will greatly enhance your yoga classes, your practice and your personal benefits.

Breath

A second concept involves the breath. Using your breath gives you energy and contributes to your control. Inhale when the body is opening or expanding and exhale when contracting. Breathe normally while in the holding phase of the asana. Keeping your breath connected to the physical movement helps keep the oxygen intake elevated so the muscles will be comfortable with the exercise task you are asking them to perform. The following yoga poses will be described with a breathing pattern to fit the movement. You will be using the Ujjayi breathing technique which is explained in detail in Unit 5. where the benefits of the various yoga breathing techniques are discussed.

Counterpose

A third concept that is an integral part of doing yoga, is to use a "counterpose" to balance the body. For example, if you have done a pose that contracts the muscles of the back, then you follow with a pose that will gently stretch that muscle group. This can apply to all areas of the body. Muscle imbalance can be the cause of postural aches and pains. Hatha yoga helps bring this situation to your attention. You will become aware of habits of sitting, standing and walking which you may want to change or improve. Let this new awareness of your postural alignment spill over into your daily living

PREPARATION POSES

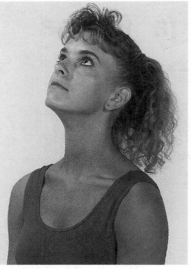

Figure 3.1   *Neck Stretch*

Neck Stretch

Benefits: Improves the range of motion in the neck.
Precautions: Go very slowly if you have problems in the cervical vertebrae. Do not FORCE.
Directions: Sitting with back erect, gently bring the chin to the chest then lift the head up to gaze at ceiling. Do NOT drop head back.
Breath: Inhale as lower and exhale as raise.

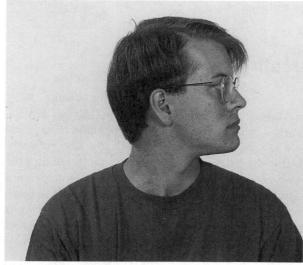

Figure 3.2   *Neck Turn*

Neck Turn

Benefits: Improvers the range of motion in the neck.
Precautions: Go very slowly if you have problems in the cervical vertebrae. Do Not FORCE.
Directions: Sitting with back erect gently turn the head from side to side noting that it is kept level and how far you are able to turn comfortably before feeling resistance. Notice also a possible difference from the right and left sides.
Breath: Inhale as you turn to side and **exhale** as you return to the center.

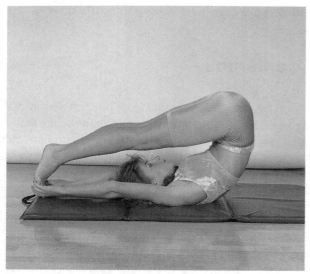

Figure 3.3   *Body Rolls*

Body Rolls

Benefits: Gently stretches the back, shoulders and legs.
Precautions: If you have injured your neck do not roll-back too far. Do gently on a padded surface. This could aggravate a past injury to the tailbone.
Directions:
1. Sitting with knees bent and hands holding the back of the thighs, roll back up onto your shoulders and then rock back up. Repeat.
2. With knees bent, set your heels on mat and reach between your legs to hold your toes. Fold your **right** leg in toward the body and then the **left** leg and lean forward, rock back as before and unfold your legs gently stretching them. Fold the legs back and rock up. Repeat folding the **left** leg in first. Laugh if you want! Classes always do.
Breath: Inhale. Exhale as roll back, **inhale** as you rock forward.

Knee Thigh Stretch (Bhadrasana)

Benefits: Improves the flexibility of the hip and knee.

Precautions: Be careful if you have injured your knees.

Directions: Sit with back erect and soles of feet together, forearms placed on thighs. Gently press down untilyou feel a gentle stretching and then hold for 10 seconds. Repeat. Notice where your legs are in relation to the mat and notice how tight or flexible you feel.

Breath: Breathe normally.

Recommendations: If possible sit with the buttocks on a folded blanket or mat. This opens the angle at the hip joint and allows the back to be more erect. This is sometimes called the "butterfly".

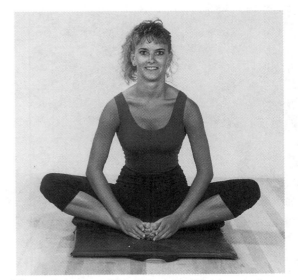

Figure 3.4 *Knee Thigh Stretch (Bhadrasana)*

One Knee to Chest

Benefits: Improves the flexibility of the back, knee and hip. Also known as the gas reliever pose.

Precautions: Place hand on the thigh behind the lower leg and knee.

Directions: Lie on back, bending the **right** knee and draw the bent leg toward the chest. Change to the **left** leg and repeat.

Breath: Inhale and then **exhale** as bring leg to chest, breath normally as you hold the stretch and **inhale** as straighten leg.

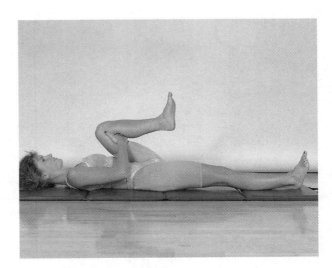

Figure 3.5 *One Knee to Chest*

Diagonal Knee to Chest

Benefits: Provides a gentle stretch for the piriformis muscle.

Precautions: Place the hand on the thigh behind the lower leg and knee.

Directions: Lie on back, bending the **right** knee and draw the bent leg diagonally across the chest toward the **left** shoulder. If the piriformis muscle is tight you will feel the stretch in the buttock area. Repeat wth the **left** leg.

Breath: Inhale and then **exhale** as you bring the leg to the chest - breathing normally as you hold the stretch. **Inhale** as you straighten and lower the leg.

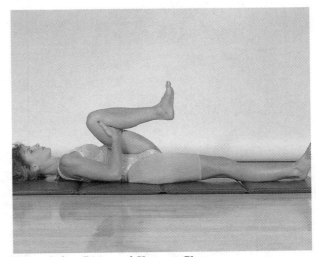

Figure 3.6 *Diagonal Knee to Chest*

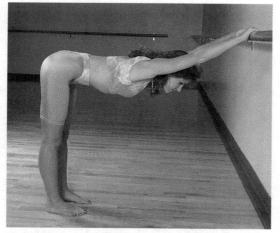

Figure 3.7   *Shoulder & Back Stretch at Wall or
Ballet Barre*

Shoulder & Back Stretch at Wall or Ballet Barre

Benefits: Marvelous stretch for the spine, arms, shoulders, muscles of the ribcage and waist area and legs.

Precautions: None.

Directions: Stand facing the wall, barre, or a counter top and have your hands holding there as you back away placing the feet directly under the hips and apart. Back should be horizontal, arms straight, neck relaxed, and shoulders are pulled toward spine. Feel the opening in the front of the chest, armpits, shoulders and the lengthening of the spine. Contract the abdominal muscles. You also may feel a stretch in the legs.

Breath: Breathe normally.

Thigh Toner

Benefits: Strengthens the quadriceps and the muscles of feet, and improves balance.

Precautions: Do not lower too far and cause stress on the knee.

Directions: Stand erect in good postural alignment and with toes spread raise on to them and balance as you lower body slightly. Keep the shoulders relaxed and over the hips. Hold as you count to 10 and then increase count as you gain more control.

Breath: Breathe normally. Watch for a tendency to hold the breath.

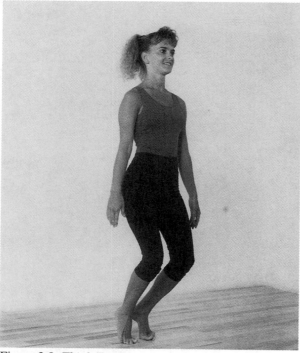

Figure 3.8 *Thigh Toner*

Head Lift & Turn

Benefits: Strengthens muscles of the neck especially the sternocleidomastoid.

Precautions: Do not do if you have had a recent neck injury.

Directions: Lying on the back, lift head an inch from the mat and hold for 6 counts, turn head to the **right** and hold for 6 counts, turn head to the **left** and hold for 6 counts, back to center and lower. Massage front of neck. Increase the count by 2 every lesson.

Breath: Breathe normally.

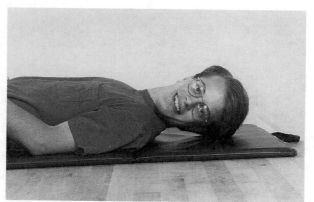

Figure 3.9 *Head Lift & Turn*

Feldenkrais Kneeovers

Benefits: Gently stretches the musclesof rib cage, back, hips, chest and neck.

Precautions: Do gently, slowly and do not force any body parts- let gravity help.

Directions: Lie on your back with knees bent, **right** leg over the **left** and **left** foot on floor. Arms should be straight out to the side from the shoulder. Lower the legs to the **right** and turn the head to look at the **left** hand. Hold. Switch the legs and repeat to the other side.

Breath: Take deep breaths and allow body to relax into the stretch.

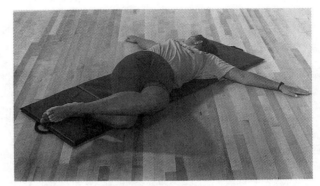

Figure 3.10 *Feldenkrais Kneeovers*

Toe-Hold Leg Lift

Benefits: Improves flexibility of the knees,ankles and hips, and stretches hamstrings.

Precautions: Be careful if you have injured the hamstring.

Directions:

1. **With Necktie.** Sitting on the mat, bend the knee and place necktie under the ball of the foot. While holding the ends of the tie straighten the leg and slowly raise until you feel a gentle stretch. Try not to lean back and away from your stretch. Hold, and lower slowly and repeat with other leg.

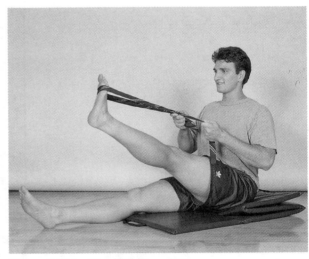

Figure 3.11A *Toe-Hold Leg Lift*

2. **Holding Toes.** Bend knee and while holding toes gently straighten the leg and draw the leg closer to the body without leaning back. When the stretch is felt hold at that position and gently lower the leg to the mat.

Breath: Breathe normally.

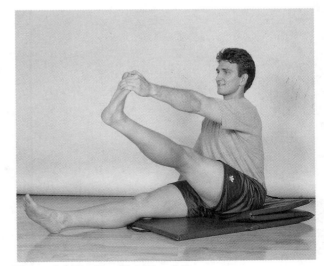

Figure 3.11B *Toe-Hold Leg Lift*

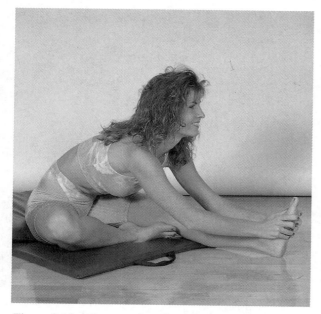

Figure 3.12 *Alternate Leg Stretch (Janusasana)*

Alternate Leg Stretch (Janusasana)

Benefits: Improves flexibility of the legs, back, and hip joints.

Precautions: Don't over stretch - go gently. Think of the muscles as rubberbands and control the stretch from beginning to end.

Directions:
1. **With necktie.** While sitting on the mat with the **left** leg extended slightly to the **left** and the **right** leg bent with the sole of **right** foot next to the **left** thigh, place necktie around the ball of the **left** foot and hold in both hands. With back erect, shoulders down from ears, lead with your sternum to bring chest closer to your **left** thigh. Do NOT drop head but gaze forward. Hold in your stretch. Repeat with the other leg.
2. Sitting in the same position as described above. Place your hands on your shoulders and reach up, straightening arms and lifting rib cage. Contract the abdominals and move forward from the hip joint. Head should be up, and shoulders away from the ears. Slowly bring your hands down to the lower leg. Note how the stretch feels in this position. If you want to increase the stretch move the hands closer to the feet. If you want to decrease the stretch move the hands closer to the knee. Hold and repeat with other leg.

Breath: Inhale as you lift up lengthening the spine and **exhale** as you fold forward.

ASANAS

Mountain Pose (Tadasana)

Benefits: Improves posture and strengthens feet

Precautions: Don't lock the knees or allow the head to drop back.

Directions: Stand erect in bare feet, facing a mirror if possible. Legs are directly under the hips. Contract quadricep and abdominal muscles. Tuck the pelvis under and lift the chest. The head is balanced over the spine. Slowly raise the arms so they are beside the ears and fingers are straight but relaxed and pointing toward the ceiling with the palms facing each other. Let the shoulders be relaxed downward and back.

Breath: **Inhale** deeply as the arms raise - the rib cage also lifts thus expanding more. Breathe full and deep while you hold the pose. **Exhale** as you lower the arms to your sides.

Recommendations: When doing the mountain pose be aware of the strength of the feet and legs supporting you and a feeling of being "grounded" as a mountain is "grounded" in the earth. Also be aware of the lightness of the arms and rib cage as they are reaching up to the sky just as a mountain peak reaches into the clouds. Feel the spine lengthening. If you are working in front of a mirror, check to see if your shoulders and the hips are level, both feet are pointed straight ahead, and that your weight is evenly placed on both feet. Stand sideways to a mirror and check for an erect back with the shoulders not overly rounded (kyphosis), and the rear end not protruding too much with a large curve in the lumbar spine (lordosis). The abdomen should be lifted. The head should not be forward of the spine as this increases the weight of the head and causes muscle fatigue. When you have the skeleton of the body lined up directly over the feet and the bones are bearing the weight as they are designed to, there is less work for the muscles, tendons and ligaments. Be aware at all times of your overall posture - whether you are standing or sitting. This standing position of the Mountain Pose is the base for all of the standing poses that will follow.

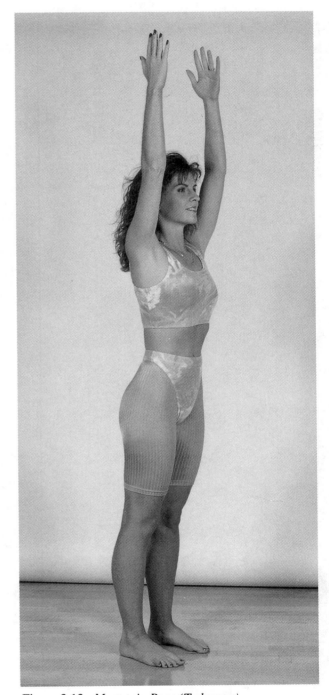

Figure 3.13 *Mountain Pose (Tadasana)*

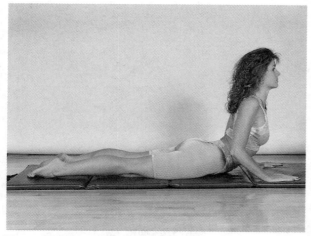

Figure 3.14A *Cobra (Bhujangasana)*

Cobra (Bhujangasana)

Benefits: Strengthens the muscles of the back and gently stretches the spine.

Precautions: Do not do if you have injured your spine recently. This is done slowly and with control. Do not tilt head back.

Directions: Lie on the abdomen with the hands placed under the shoulders, and the forehead resting on the mat. Move the head by brushing the chin across the mat. Contract the abdominal muscles, thus lifting the navel from the mat. Slowly bring the chest up off the mat. Use the muscles of the back to lift the torso rather than pushing up with the arms. Keep the abdominal muscles engaged as you slowly lower the chest back to mat. Repeat twice.

Breath: **Inhale** as you lift up into the pose and **exhale** as you lower back to the mat, tucking the chin.

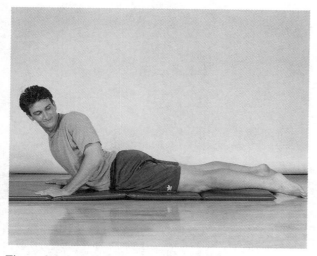

Figure 3.14B *Cobra with Head Turn*

Variation: Cobra with Head Turn

Directions: Separate the legs slightly, lift into the cobra following the above directions. **Exhale** and as you stay in the Cobra **inhale** as you turn the head to gaze over the **right** shoulder at the **right** heel and **exhale** as you return the head to face forward. **Inhale** and turn the head slowly to the **left** to gaze over the **left** shoulder at the **left** heel and **exhale** as you return to the center. **Inhale** and **exhale** as you lower to starting position.

Recommendations: This pose needs to be done with control and executed slowly. When in the pose, the chin is lifted slightly and the gaze is slightly up - do NOT tilt the head back and compress the cervical verte-brae. The imagery here is of a snake moving slowly, with great flexibility and fluidity of movement. Don't hunch the shoulders by the ears and don't worry about straightening the arms. Be aware of the spine and the muscles of the back contracting. Always do a COUNTERPOSE of either the FETUS or KNEES TO CHEST pose.

Half Locust
(Ardha Salabhasana)

Benefits: Strengthens muscles of back, rear end and legs.

Precautions: Do not do if you have injured the lower back or have a chronic problem. If you have a problem with the sciatic nerve, be cautious as you try this. Do the asana slowly and do not lift the leg very high.

Directions: Lie on abdomen, with hands beside thighs, palms facing down. Place chin on the mat to keep the head straight. IMPORTANT: contract abdominal muscles - lifting the navel from the mat. Contract muscles of **right** leg and lift leg slowly upward to the point you are comfortable. Hold and then lower with control. Do the **left** leg and repeat 2 more times with each leg. Practice this pose with the foot flexed and push the heel away from you noticing how the muscles in the buttocks become engaged.

Breath: **Inhale** as you lift the leg and hold, **exhale** as you lower.

Recommendations: Do not stay in the pose for too long and risk not being able to control the lowering. Always do the COUNTERPOSE of FETUS or KNEES TO CHEST.

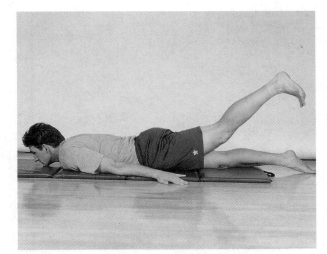

Figure 3.15 *Half Locust (Ardha Salabhasana)*

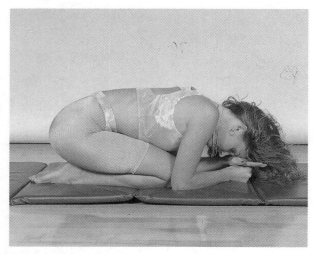

Figure 3.16A   *Fetus*

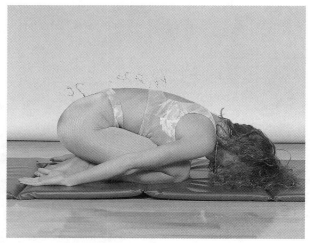

Figure 3.16B   *Fetus*

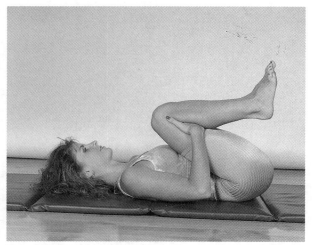

Figure 3.17   *Knees to Chest*

Fetus

Benefits: Gently stretches the entire back, relaxes the neck, and improves flexibility in the legs, ankles and feet.

Precautions: May be uncomfortable if you have problems with injured knees or ankles. If so do the KNEES to CHEST pose following.

Directions: Kneeling, place hips on the heels and keep them there as you lower the head to the mat in several stages that will be described. If the hips leave the heels STOP at that position and rest in the pose. The head will be resting on the hands as they will change position - do the hand positions first:

1. Hands in fists one on top of the other
2. Top hand flattens out and is on top of bottom hand
3. Two hands make fists and go side by side
4. Two hands flatten - one on top of the other
5. Two hands slide apart to be side by side
6. Two hands slide clear apart for head to be on mat.
7. Move arms to rest on mat beside the legs allowing shoulders to fully relax

Breath: Breathe normally as you relax and let go.

Recommendations: Always do this pose to gently stretch the muscles of the back after they havebeen contracted. Also, do at any time when thereis the feeling of tightness or fatigue in low back-such as after wearing high heels or standing for a prolonged time. You can also rest the forehead on a pillow.

Knees to Chest

Benefits: Gently stretches the back. This is an optional counterpose when the back muscles have been contracted.

Precautions: Do not place hands on lower legs.

Directions: Lie on back and bring both knees to the chest with hands on the thighs behind the knees. Gently hug self feeling a gentle stretch in the back. Lifting the head will increase the stretch.

Breath: Breathe normally as you relax into stretch.

Recommendations: Do this pose when there is a problem with the knees or ankles that makes kneeling in the fetus pose uncomfortable.

Sitting Forward Bend (Paschimottansana)

Benefits: Improves flexibility of hamstrings, hips, and back and also lengthens spine.

Precautions: Don't overstretch.

Directions: Sitting with legs out straight in front of you and back erect, place a necktie around balls of the flexed feet. Contract abdominal muscles and bend forward at the hip joint - lead with the sternum and keep the shoulders back and head up. Feel the stretch in the hamstrings and the back. Now bend the knees to take the stretch off the hamstrings. Lower your self further, feeling the stretch more in the back. Repeat two more times.

Breath: Inhale as you lead with sternum and **exhale** as you fold forward at the hip joint. Breath normally as you relax into the stretch. **Inhale** as you lift up and **exhale** as you fold forward on your repeats.

Recommendations: Notice how far forward you moved into the pose before you felt the stretch so you can be aware of your progress. Notice also where you felt the tightness - legs or back. Do sideways to a mirror if possible to better note your progress. Also this pose can be done without the necktie when you have learned to keep a good alignment in the back - you place the hands on the lower legs, ankles or feet - where ever is comfortable (Fig. 3.18B).

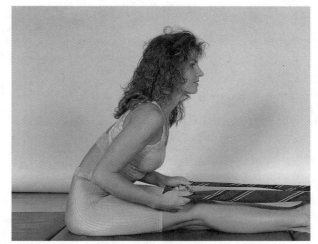

Figure 3.18A   *Sitting Forward Bend (Paschimottansana)*

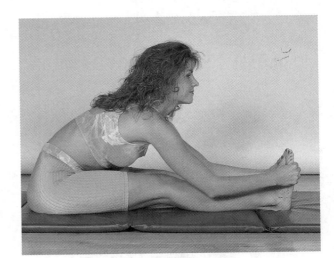

Figure 3.18B   *Sitting Forward Bend (Paschimottansana)*

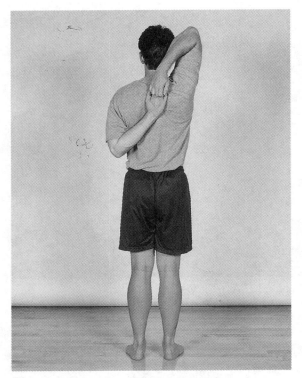

Figure 3.19A   *Head of Cow (Gomukhasana)*

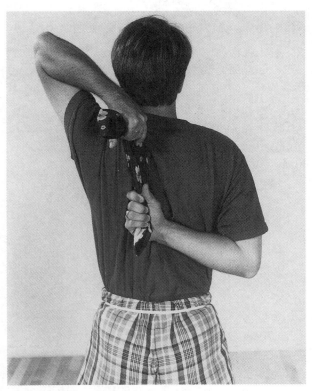

Figure 3.19B   *Head of Cow (Gomukhasana)*

Head of Cow (Gomukhasana)

Benefits: Gently stretches the muscles of the shoulders and arms. Improves posture.

Precautions: Be cautious if you have injured your wrist, elbow or shoulder. Do not force yourself into the pose.

Directions: Stand erect, and raise **right** arm so the upper arm is by your ear and you can pat yourself on your back when you bend your elbow. Bring your **left** arm behind you with the palm facing out and placed as high on your back as you can reach. Do your hands touch? Can you join your fingers together? If so-congratulations! If not, use the necktie (Fig 3.19B) and drop it down your back with the **left** hand and grasp it with the **right** hand. Now that you are joined gently pull down with the **left** hand and gently pull up with the **right** hand and as you do so you will feel a gentle response in your arms and shoulders. Repeat, reversing arms.

Breath: Breathe normally. Do NOT hold breath.

Recommendations: Notice the ease in which you are able to join your hands or how far apart your hands are if you are using the neck tie. You may be able to do it on one side but not on the other. Position shoulders over the hips with the spine straight - avoid arching the back and pushing the abdomen forward. With daily practice you will make progress and be able to see and feel your improvement. A good time to practice is when you are showering and have the washcloth or towel to use in place of the necktie. Do not let anyone "HELP" you by pushing your hands closer together!. Look over your shoulder in a mirror to see your progress. Try doing the arm positions when:

1. Kneeling on your lower legs
2. Sitting with the weight on the lower **right** leg with the **right** foot back beside the **left** buttock; the **left** leg crosses over the **right** knee and the **left** heel back by the **right** thigh or hip. Reverse the leg position.

Chest Expansion
(Araha Chakrasana)

Benefits: Gently stretches the pectoral muscles, improves posture, prevents kyphosis (round shoulders), brings blood to face and brain, stretches out the muscles in the neck, improves flexibility of elbows and wrists, and perks you up when feeling sluggish.

Precautions: Don't do if you have glaucoma, cataract surgery or a problem with the retina of the eyes. If you have high or low blood pressure do not stay in the position with the head down very long and come up slowly. Please check with your physician if brain cancer is present or if you have had a recent injury to the head.

Directions: Stand in the MOUNTAIN POSE (sideways to a mirror if possible),bring hands up to front of chest and extend arms straight out in front of you. Without allowing torso to move, separate the arms, move them out to the side keeping them at shoulder height bringing the hands together and interlocking the fingers behind you. STRAIGHTEN the arms and notice the marvelous stretch in the front of the chest. Now slowly bend forward allowing the arms to lift up and point toward the ceiling. (If by a mirror-glance to see the arm position and how much space there is between your arms and your back). Allow:

1. The torso to fold at the hip hinge keeping the hips over the feet;
2. Gravity to lengthen the spine;
3. The chest to come toward the thighs. With the head hanging free, gently allow the head to make small circles, reverse the circles, and then come up slowly. Release the hand and enjoy the feeling of exhilaration! Repeat.

Breath: Inhale as you move arms back and **exhale** as you bend forward and breath normally while you circle the head. **Inhale** as you come up and **exhale** as you end the pose and lower arms.

Recommendations: Always do slowly. If the stretch on the hamstrings is more than you are enjoying, bend the knees. If you feel that you are getting dizzy - come up immediately but slowly.

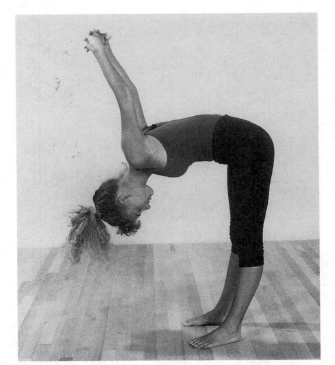

Figure 3.20   *Chest Expansion (Araha Chakrasana)*

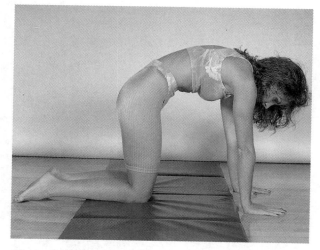

Figure 3.21A   *Cat*

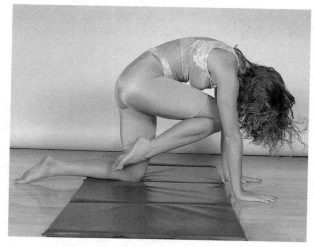

Figure 3.21B   *Variation: Cat With Leg*

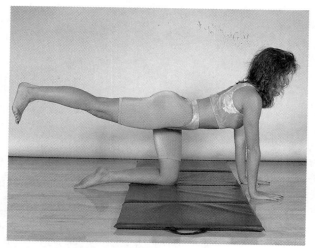

Figure 3.21C   *Variation: Cat With Leg*

Cat

Benefits: Improves flexibility of the back and hips. Strengthens the arms and shoulders.

Precautions: Knee problems can make kneeling uncomfortable. Have knees on a mat and hands on floor.

Directions: Kneeling (side to mirror if possible), place your palms, with fingers spread and pointing forward. Or for greater stability and comfort with the elbows have the **right** index finger points toward 11 o'clock and the **left** index finger is pointing toward 1 o'clock. In either position the hands are directly under the shoulders. Make sure the insides of your elbows are facing each other. Your knees are directly under the hips with space between them. Contract the abdominal muscles. Lift your rounded back up toward the ceiling like a cat. Allow the head to drop forward. Then lower the back until it sags, lifting the head. Repeat several times.

Variation: Cat With Leg As the back lifts, bring a bent knee into the chest, as the back lowers, extend the leg back so that the heel is in line with the buttocks and the shoulder. The foot should be flexed and the head lifted up as you gaze forward. Repeat with other leg and do two more with each leg (Fig. 3.21 B & C).

Breath: Inhale and then **exhale** as back lifts and/or knee comes in toward chest and then **inhale** as head lifts and leg is extended.

Recommendations: Be aware of the abdominal area - don't let it sag. When the leg movement is added, do not let the heel be higher than the hip, thus insuring that the lumbar area of the back is not compressed. Be aware of any possible differences between the **right** and **left** leg as they come forward. Keep fingers flat and pressed to the floor with the elbows in proper alignment. When you have finished, shake your hands to release any tension in your wrists.

Variation: Cat "Push-Up and Down"

Benefits: Strengthens the arms and shoulders, improves flexibility in the joints.

Precautions: Don't do if have a recent injury to wrist, shoulders or elbows.

Directions: Kneeling on all fours, (place the knees on mat or folded blanket and the hands and feet on the floor) turn the **right** index finger to point at 11 o'clock and the **left** index finger to point at 1 o'clock. Keep the shin bones and hands pressing downward. Lift abdominal muscles. Lower the chest toward the floor between the arms. The bent elbows move outwards. Lift up, pressing to floor with the hands and the shin bones of the lower legs, rounding the spine upward and taking the hips back to the heels, allowing a stretch through the back. Lift up to all fours. Repeat with a continuous flowing motion.

Breath: Inhale in starting pose, **exhale** as lower chest to floor. **Inhale** while lifting up and moving hips to heels. **Exhale** while allowing stretch to happen. **Inhale** while lifting to all fours and **exhale** while lowering chest. Repeat 4-8 times.

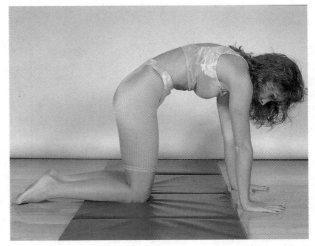

Figure 3.22A   *Variation: Cat "Push-Up and Down"*

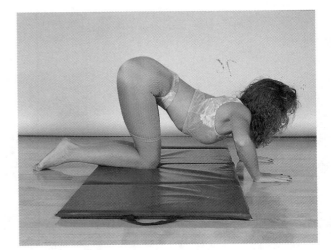

Figure 3.22B   *Variation: Cat "Push-Up and Down"*

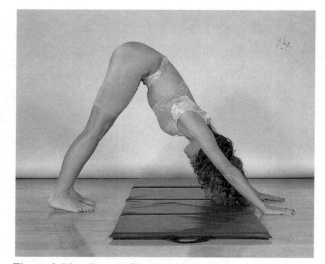

Figure 3.23   *Dog (Adho Mukha Svanasana)*

Dog (Adho Mukha Svanasana)

Benefits: Improves flexibility in the legs (especially the gastrocnemius) and shoulders, as well as lengthening the spine and strengthening the shoulders and arms. It is also an inverted pose which brings the blood to the face and brain, thus benefiting that area without putting any strain on the muscles of the neck.

Precautions: Do not do if you have glaucoma or retina problems or recent eye surgery. Do not stay long if you have high or low blood pressure. If you have injured the achilles tendon be cautious when allowing the stretch to move into that area. Must be done in bare feet on the floor.

Directions: Starting position is the "all fours " used in the CAT "Pushup & Down" with all the same directions for achieving a good alignment. Adjust the hands to turn slightly inward. Turn under the toes and use them to grip the floor while lifting the buttocks toward the ceiling. Keep arms straight and press to floor with hands to better elongate the spine. BE STRONG. Lower your heels to the floor as far as you are comfortable . Bend your knees slightly, lowering the heels one at a time toward the floor. Lower the knees to the mat and relax.

Breath: Inhale deeply before beginning and then keep the breath deep and regular as you hold in the pose. Do not hold the breath as the breath helps you to stay energized and to be strong in the pose.

Recommendations: Don't ever force. Think STRONG.Don't move the hands and feet from the starting alignment position. Do sideways to a mirror to see if you are achieving an upside down "V" position with the asana. Keep the energy moving downward to the hands and feet and upward with the buttocks.

Yoga Sit Back & Up

Benefits: Strengthens even very weak abdominal muscles in the sitting back phase.

Precautions: Could aggravate an injured tailbone or a hernia. Don't do immediately after abdominal surgery.

Directions: Do sitting on a mat with the back erect and knees bent. Contract the abdominal muscles firmly. While holding them contracted throughout the movement pattern lower your back-

1. To a 45° angle and hold
2. Until you are on your sacrum and hold
3. Until the shoulders are barely on the mat and hold
4. Release the contraction, and stretch the arms and legs while taking a deep breath
5. If you have strong abdominal muscles you will come up reversing the procedure
6. If your muscles are weak, roll over on to your side and repeat the going down phase.

Breath: Breathe normally. Do not hold the breath. Breathe shallowly in the top part of the lung when the abdomen is contracted.

Recommendations: Follow this pose with a gentle COBRA to gently stretch the abdominal muscles. Do this pose daily if your abdominal muscles are weak. Make sure you get a strong contraction before you move to the holding stages. Do 2-3 times. To increase the work load you can move the arms out to the side or above your head.

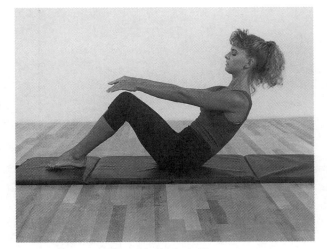

Figure 3.24A   *Yoga Sit Back & Up*

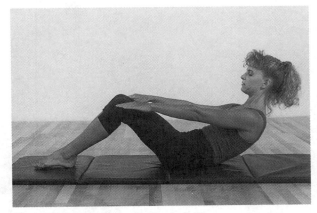

Figure 3.24B   *Yoga Sit Back & Up*

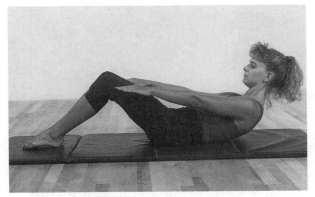

Figure 3.24C   *Yoga Sit Back & Up*

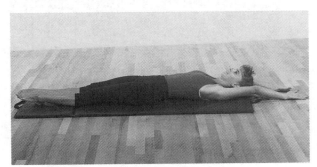

Figure 3.24D   *Yoga Sit Back & Up*

Shoulderstand (Sarvangasana)

Benefits: In Sanskrit the word SARVA means "all" and the word ANGA means "parts." The name implies that this pose is for all body parts - thus there are many benefits. Being an inverted pose it allows the body to overcome some of the effects of gravity on the veins, arteries, and internal organs by placing the body in an opposite alignment. This can be helpful for a prolapsed uterus. The circulation to the legs, spine, thyroid gland and brain is enhanced by this pose. Those with asthma and throat problems also benefit from doing this pose. The muscles of the back and shoulders are strengthened. The pose is energizing.

Precautions: The major precautions will be discussed under the variations section as they will vary depending on individuals needs. In general, however, this pose is not recommended for those with high blood pressure or recent neck injuries. If you are menstruating or are pregnant do the variation in Fig 3.25A that is described below.

Directions: Will be given for each variation.

Variations:

A. **Fig. 3.25A** At the wall simply elevate the legs and be aware of the feeling in the legs as the circulation is affected by this position.

　Recommendations: This variation can be done by almost everyone. This especially should be done by those women who are pregnant or are having their menstrual cycle. This position is also safe for someone who has injured their neck, has high blood pressure, a hernia, or is 20-30 pounds overweight.

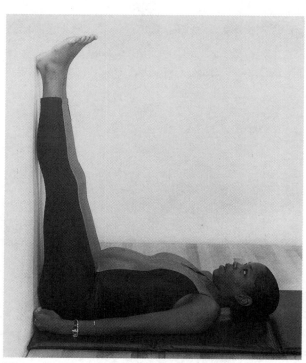

Figure 3.25A   *Shoulderstand (Sarvangasana)*

B. **Fig. 3.25B** Start in the position described above invariation "A". Bend the knees, walk the feet up the wall and support the back with the hands. The body will now be in a slant with a little more weight placed on the shoulders. Take one leg away from the wall at a time to get the feel for balancing. Then take both legs away and hold in a half shoulderstand position.

Precautions: Do not do if pregnant or menstruating.

Recommendations: When you are feeling comfortable in this position you are ready to work with the next variation. Remember this variation is not recommemded if you are pregnant or menstruating. Follow with the FISH for your counterpose.

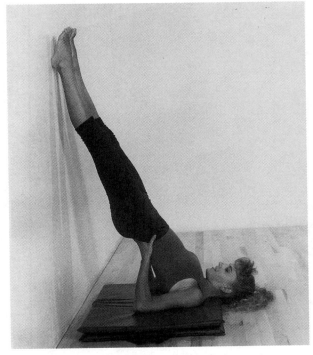

Figure 3.25B   *Shoulderstand (Sarvangasana)*

C. **Fig 3.25C On Folded Blanket or Folded Yoga Mat**
Fold either a solid blanket or a mat so it is about one to two inches thick. Lie on the mat with the edge of the shoulders about one inch away from the edge of the folded mat or blanket. The head should be resting on the floor and with air or space between the cervical vertebrae and the floor below.This allows the neck to maintain its natural curve and does not hyperflex the neck and over stretch the supporting muscles. It is nice to have a partner stand by your head to assist you with the alignment and to help guide you as you bring your knees to your chest, lift up your lower back and support it with your hands. Now that you are up, you are ready to do some fine-tuning with your asana. Bring your shoulders toward the spine - squeezing them together. Slowly extend your legs up, tightening the buttocks and hamstrings. Imagine that your spine is straight. Hold in the pose 1 to 2 minutes, eventually working up to 4-5 minutes. Keep adjusting the rotation of the shoulder blades to the spine if you feel them losing the alignment. Remember to do the FISH. as a counterpose.

Precautions: Do <u>not</u> do this variation and the one following if you are pregnant, menstruating, have high blood pressure, a hernia, neck injury or are 20-30 pounds over your desirable weight. Also be careful if you are overtired or are recovering from an illness.

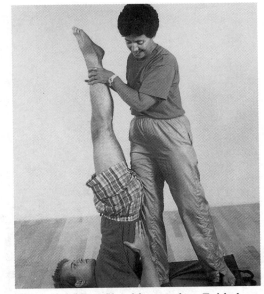

Figure 3.25C   *Shoulderstand on Folded Blanket or Yoga Mat*

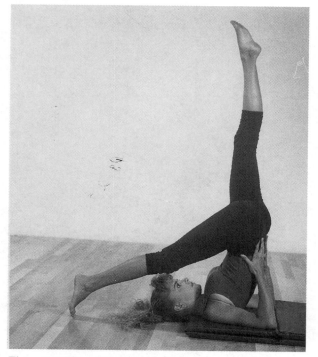

Figure 3.25D   *Shoulderstand with Leg Movements*

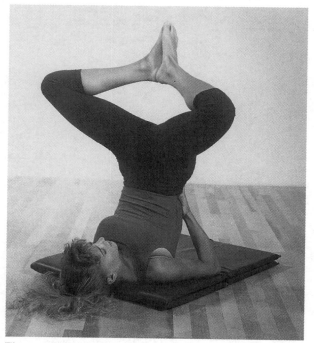

Figure 3.25E   *Shoulderstand with Leg Movements*

Fig 3.25 D & E   Leg movements Do these when you are able to stay centered and balanced with back erect in VARIATION C.

1. Split the legs apart into a wide "V." Hold. While the legs are in the "V," move them slowly from front to back allowing a gentle twist to occur thus stretching the muscles of the back.
2. Lower the **right** toe to the floor behind your head and keep the **left** foot reaching toward the ceiling. Lift the **right** foot up and repeat with the **left** foot. (Fig. 3.25D)
3. Place the soles of the feet together and draw the heels down toward the crotch with the knees out to the side. You will look like you are a frog! (Fig. 3.25E)

Recommendations: Never turn your head, and always come down with control having your hands support your back until it is strong enough to uncurl. Keep the back of the head on the floor as you are rolling down out of the shoulderstand. Always do the COUNTER POSE of the FISH and the CHEST EXPANSION to balance the body. If you experience some muscle twinges of fatigue in the back muscles, it will most likely disappear after the FISH, and as your back muscles become stronger.

Breath: Keep the breath flowing at all times in all of the variations. As the abdominal muscles become stronger the feeling of pressure against your diaphragm will lessen. When you have come down out of your shoulderstand, take some deep breaths.

Fish (Matsyasana)

Benefits: This pose is used as a counterpose to balance the body following the shoulderstand as it places the body in an opposite position. For example, the neck which had the chin to the chest is now being stretched with the head going back; the front of the chest was semi-cramped and in this pose it is opened up; and the back muscles had been strengthened and stretched and are now going to be contracted ridding you of any muscles tension you may be experiencing. It is also very beneficial for the nasal passages and the sinuses as the circulation is increased to the area. When you raise the head you may notice drainage in the back of the throat. This pose also strengthens the muscles of the neck.

Precautions: Do not cough, swallow, laugh or sneeze while in the fish pose as your neck is in a vulnerable position. If you are susceptible to motion sickness or have an inner ear disturbance you may experience dizziness. If you have high blood pressure don't stay in the pose very long. This pose could also aggravate an old neck injury so be cautious as you try it your first time.

Directions: Lie on your back and place your hands, palm down, under your buttocks. Raise up so that you are leaning back on your lower arms and elbows. Imagine lifting your sternum toward the ceiling and, while maintaining the arch in your back, slowly lean back until the top of the head is resting on the mat. Stay in this position for 4-5 deep breaths and as you exhale the last one lift the head up and sit up OR if the head feels very heavy (it actually weighs from 10-15 lbs.) slide your hands out from under you and lower your back to the mat.

Breath: **Inhale** as deeply as you can through your nose allowing the chest to expand as fully as possible.

Recommendations: Do this pose daily if you are prone to nasal congestion or sinus problems. Always do following the SHOULDERSTAND.

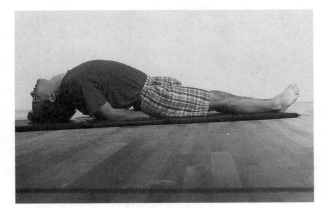

Figure 3.26   *Fish (Matsyasana)*

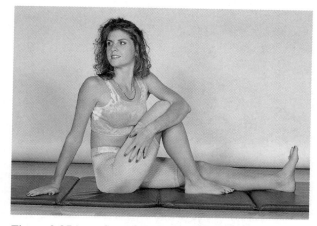

Figure 3.27A   *Spinal Twist (Ardha Matsyendrasana)*

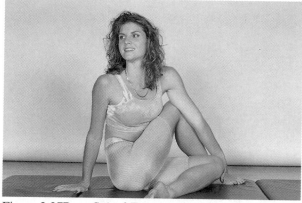

Figure 3.27B   *Spinal Twist (Ardha Matsyendrasana)*

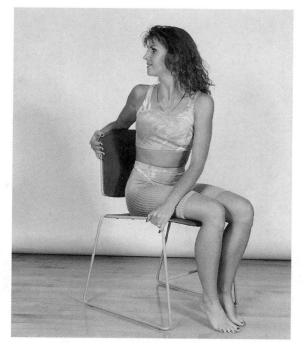

Figure 3.27C   *Spinal Twist (Ardha Matsyendrasana)*

Spinal Twist (Ardha Matsyendrasana)

Benefits: Improves greatly the flexibility of the spine. Helps you become aware of your ability to turn equally to both sides. Gentle warm-up for all the muscles of the back. Improves breathing capacity.

Precautions: Do not do if you have a herniated spinal disc. Be gentle with yourself if you have any other injuries to your back or neck.

Directions: Sit with back erect and both legs out straight in front of you. Bend the **right** leg, place the foot on the mat on the outside of the **left** knee with the **right** knee pointing toward the ceiling. Place your hands on top of the **right** knee and do a gentle turn to your **right** and to your left to warm up the back. Now lift the **right** arm upward in an arc, placing the palm on the floor behind the **right** buttock. The **left** arm is placed on the outside of the **right** thigh or knee applying some leverage as your head now turns to look over the **right** shoulder. Hold in the position as you count to 10. Repeat with the twist going to the **left**.

Breath: You breathe in a normal fashion in this pose. With the leg pressing next to the chest it is difficult to get a full deep breath as you are turning. Do NOT hold the breath- keep it flowing.

Recommendations: Keep the head level as it turns. Imagine the spine is a corkscrew and you are gradually turning the spine in that fashion as the twist progresses. Move your back hand to a new position if you feel you could twist further. Maintain a straight spine with no backward lean with the torso. Always remember that the opposite arm goes by the opposite leg for the maximun twist.

Variation: The leg that is out straight can be bent and the foot brought back under the opposite buttock. The arm by the leg can be straightened and the hand placed on the ankle. The arm that is back can be placed around waist. Eventually, with practice, the two hands can join under the bent knee.

Tree (Vriksasana)

Benefits: Strengthens the feet and the legs. Improves posture, balance, and flexibility of the hip and knee.

Precautions: This pose may be challenging if you have injured your foot or ankle - but don't be discouraged. To prevent falling out of balance, do the pose with a hand placed on a wall or chair back for support.

Directions: Begin by doing the MOUNTAIN POSE without the arm lift. Place the weight on the **left** leg with the muscles contracted and holding you firm. Make small circles with the **right** leg before lifting it and placing the sole of the **right** foot on the inner **left** thigh as high as you can put it. Maintain the rest of the alignment suggestions AND your balance. The **right** knee should be facing to the side. Now for the fine tuning: Tuck the pelvis under slightly - keep the hips level and the abdominal muscles contracted. If you are steady and balanced, then start to make the arm movements: Slowly lift the arms above the head as you also lift the rib cage, but lower the shoulders. Touch the fingers together with the elbows pointing to the side. Image a TREE that is solid with its roots in the earth and its upper branches light and reaching to the sky. With control, lower the arms, then the **right** leg. Pause and center in and then repeat with the weight on the **right** leg and the **left** leg lifted to the bent position. Be aware of any differences in balance, control or alignment between the two sides as you execute the asana.

Breath: The breath is very important in this posture. **Inhale** and then **exhale** as you make your movements. While holding in the pose breath deeply and keep the breath flowing so that you maintain energy and control.

Recommendations: It helps tremendously to FOCUS on something that is not moving. Chose a spot on the floor or the wall in front of you. Try closing your eyes while in the TREE and see what happens. WHOOPS! Hope you didn't fall! Remember to be steady at one stage before you make your movement to the next position. This pose can be practiced while talking on the phone, doing dishes, washing your face, or standing in line.

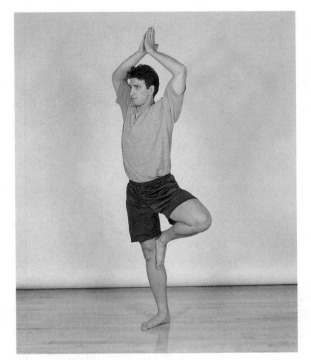

Figure 3.28   *Tree (Vriksasana)*

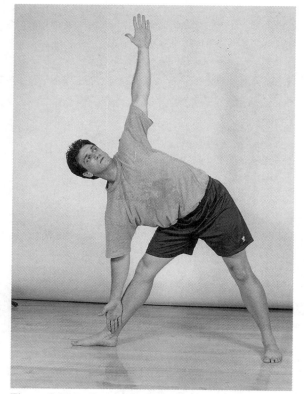

Figure 3.29   *Triangle (Trikonasana)*

Triangle (Trikonasana)

Benefits: Improves flexibility of the spine and shoulders. Stretches and strengthens the muscles of the leg. Tones the muscles of the waist, abdomen and the intercostal muscles of the ribcage which are important for deep breathing.

Precautions: You may notice fatigue in areas of old injuries such as shoulders, legs   or back when doing the pose but this will probably go away as the area gains in strength. Stop if pain is present.

Directions: Stand in the MOUNTAIN POSE and then jump to a wide stance with the feet wider than the hips (3-4' apart). As you jump out extend your arms out to the side at shoulder height. Keep pelvis facing forward and arms level. IMPORTANT - pivot on the **right** heel rotating the femur outward in the hip joint and contract the quadricep muscles to stabalize the knee. Place the **right** finger tips at the top of the **right** thigh where the leg joins at the hip hinge and lean over to the **right** side.   Now place the **right** hand behind your head and then image that you are reaching to the far wall as you extend the arm out to the **right**.   Lower your arm to rest in front of the **right** knee but DON'T let the rib cage, which you just extended, collapse. The **left** arm is straight and pointing to the ceiling. Let the neck remain soft and be extended straight from the spine. When all the above alignment corrections are made turn your head to gaze upward at the hand. To come up from the pose image that someone is holding your **left** hand and is gently lifting you up to the beginning position. Pause and reflect on what you experienced and then repeat going to the **left** side following all the above directions. Repeat 2 more times each side.

Breath: You get your energy to hold the asana from the breath. First **inhale** deeply and **exhale** as you jump to the straddle stance. **Inhale** as you turn the leg and then **exhale** as you lower into the position. Breathe deeply while holding the asana. When ready to come up, **inhale** and then **exhale** as you lift back to the beginning position. **Inhale** and **exhale** here as you reflect. **Inhale** as you turn the other leg and **exhale** as you lower down to that side.

Recommendations: Remember to turn the foot to form a 90 degree angle with the arch of the other foot as this protects the knee. Practicing with your back to the wall helps you learn to keep your shoulders from rolling forward. Also it is helpful to practice in front of a mirror to check on the pelvis and the arm alignment. This pose **must** be done in bare feet.

Triangle Twist
(Parivritta Trikonasana)

Benefits: Same as for the TRIANGLE but as the spine rotates in this asana, it increases the flexibility and strength of the back.

Precautions: Same as for the TRIANGLE except for adding a caution for those with a back injury that required fusion of the vertebra.

Directions: Jump into the pose as described in TRIANGLE, pivot on the heel also to turn the leg on the side that you will be moving to- the **right**. Now pivot at the waist turning to the **right** and leading with your chest lean out over your leg . You will probably feel a stretch in the legs. Keep some of your weight on the back foot, which is your **left** one. Twisting, now lower the **left** hand down to some place on your **right** leg and notice where the hand is and at what spot the pose becomes un-comfortable. At this point, back off and raise the **left** hand so that you are still feeling a stretch but no pain. Turn the head slightly so that you can gaze at the **right** hand that is pointing to the ceiling with the arm straight. Pause and hold the asana. Move the arms until they are straight out from the shoulders. Raise the trunk and pivot back to face the front. Turn your feet to the front. Repeat all the moves now going to the **left** side.

Breath: The pattern is the same as for the TRIANGLE. With the addition of the twist you may notice the chest feeling more cramped, but as you are able to become more free in the pose the chest will be able to open up more. Keep the breath flowing while in the asana.

Recommendations: Always make sure that the quadri-ceps are contracted, the foot is turned and the op-posite hand goes down on the opposite leg in this asana. Don't lean on the leg. Keep both legs straight. Don't over reach by going down too far on the leg and losing the twist. Walk around when finished and gently shake the legs to release any tension.

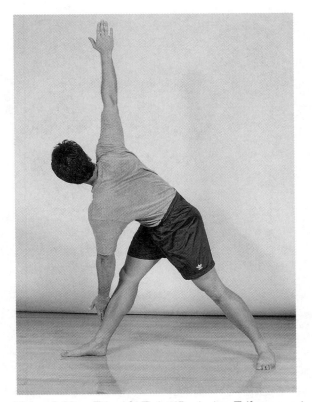

Figure 3.30   *Triangle Twist (Parivritta Trikonasana)*

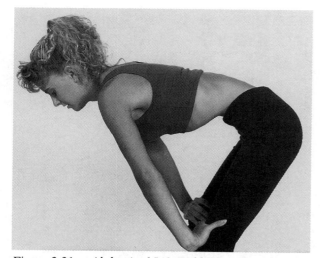

Figure 3.31   *Abdominal Lift (Uddiyana Bandha)*

Abdominal Lift (Uddiyana Bandha)

Benefits: This pose strengthens the abdominal muscles without putting any strain on the back. The circulation to the internal organs is increased and they are gently massaged. This pose is helpful for those who have a problem with constipation.

Precautions: Do not do this pose if you have: a full stomach, hernia, ulcer, recent abdominal surgery, or are pregnant. If you have a "nervous stomach" do with caution and if you think this pose causes discomfort - STOP.

Directions & Breath: Stand with knees slightly bent and palms resting on thighs just above the knees. Place your right hand on the abdomen so when you do the LIFT, you can make a comparison. Now EXHALE forcefully saying "HA." Practice this several times and feel that you are emptying your lungs as you do this. Now the tricky part - with the air exhaled, contract and lift the abdominal muscles toward the spine. Still holding, take your hand to check your abdomen. Hopefully you can feel a change and that there is a "caved in" area where your abdomen used to be. If so, you were quite successful for your first try. Don't be discouraged, as it takes practice to accomplish this but it is well worth the time spent. Hold the contraction for about 5-10 seconds and then release. Stand up and take a deep breath before you repeat. Do this about 4-5 times and do daily.

Variation: Multiple Lifts Once you have become proficient at doing the single ABDOMINAL LIFT you are ready to do this variation. When you have done your first abdominal contraction and the breath is in its suspended state, you allow the muscles to lower but NOT relax, contracting them and lifting the abdomen back up and down as many times as is comfortable, depending on your breath control. Don't do too many at first - 3 or 4. The massage on the internal organs is enhanced with this variation.

Recommendations: Practice these in the morning when the stomach is empty. If you have a problem with constipation put 1 tsp. - 1Tb. lemon juice in a glass of lukewarm water and drink this in the morning. Wait a few minutes for it to reach the stomach and then do the ABDOMINAL LIFT. This "wakes up" the digestive tract in a normal fashion. Also, it is helpful to practice this pose in front of a mirror in your underwear so that you can see what is happening and better tune into your progress. It is recommended to do this pose following childbirth when the physician has said it is time to begin to exercise. This pose is an example of a BANDHA, a type of yoga position in which a lock is placed upon the body. We get the English word "Bondage" from this Sanskrit term.

Back Push-Up (Kamaharasana)

Benefits: This pose strengthens the buttocks, thighs, abdomen and pubococygeal muscle that forms the base of the abdominal area. Having this muscle strong helps to prevent incontinence and improves the flexibility of the spine and shoulders.

Precautions: Don't lift too high and hyperflex the neck.

Directions: The pelvic tilt will be taught as it is the first step in doing this asana. Lie on your back with knees bent and slightly apart, feet flat on the floor, and hands beside the hips. Contract the abdominals and feel the lumbar area of the back press into the mat. Now arch this area up away from the mat. Place one of your hands under this arched area and tilt the pelvis down, moving the back onto your hand. Arch up, take the hand out and again do the pelvic tilt - pressing the lumbar area into the mat while contracting the abdominal muscles. Now contract the muscles of the buttocks, thighs, abdominals and the pubococygeal (the muscle you tighten when you need to go to the bathroom and there isn't one available at that moment). Lift the buttocks followed by the rest of the back from the mat. Lift until you are on the shoulders, back of head and the feet. Slowly, and with control, lower the spine one vertebra after another. Now, we will add the arm movement - as the back lifts, the arms will lift also until they are resting on the mat behind the head. Keep the pelvis lifted, hold the pose. As you lower do it slowly. Relax and take a deep breath.

Breath: Inhale as the back and the arms lift into the pose on a count of 6. Hold and breath normally and then exhale as the back and arms lower to a count of 6.

Recommendations: As a counterpose do the KNEES TO CHEST to gently stretch out the spine. This asana is a preparation for the advanced asana of the Bow, Bridge and the Wheel.

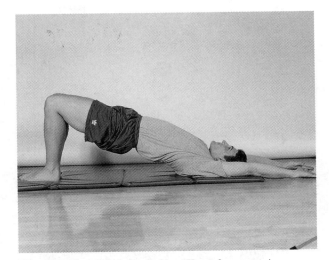

Figure 3.32   *Back Push-Up (Kamaharasana)*

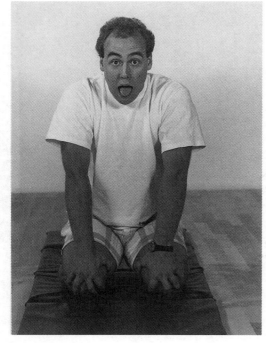

Figure 3.33 *Lion*

Lion

Benefits: Improves circulation to the throat and face. Tones the facial and throat muscles.

Precautions: Go slowly if you have a problem with the temporal mandibular joint (TMJ).

Directions: Be prepared to be uninhibited when you do this pose. You may prefer to do it in private! Kneeling (or sitting) place your hands on your knees, lean forward slightly, stick your head forward, open your mouth and eyes as wide as you can, and then stick out your tongue as far as it will go. You will look weird but it is fun to do!

Breath: You can **exhale** with a small roar if you want as you stick out the tongue.

Recommendations: This pose also warms up the vocal chords so it is recommended for singers. It also is helpful for sore throats that are caused by the irritation from post-nasal drip. Try it.

Dolphin

Benefits: Brings blood to head, thereby improving circulation to the brain. Strengthens the arms, shoulders, and back. Stretches the legs.

Precautions: Do not do if you have high blood pressure, glaucoma or retina problems, brain surgery or a recent head injury.

Directions: Kneel on a mat with your forearms on the mat and the hands interlocked. Elbows should be directly under the shoulders. Move your knees back and then place the top of your head on the mat with the joined hands snug against the back of the head. Keep the shoulders lifted away from the ears so that the neck is held strong. Straighten your legs by lifting the buttocks toward the ceiling. Hold in this inverted position. Lower down and relax with the head on the mat. Repeat. Now lift the head off the mat using the muscles of the back and the neck to do this (Fig. 3.34B). Hold - noticing how the muscles are working to help you accomplish this. Do not allow the shoulders to collapse down on to the neck.

Breath: Breathe normally as you attain the kneeling position. Then, as you straighten the legs to lift the buttocks, **exhale**. **Inhale** and **exhale** while maintaining the pose. **Exhale** while you lower buttocks down.

Recommendations: It is best to practice this after having down the CHEST EXPANSION, CAT and DOG poses. This pose is a preparation pose for the HEADSTAND HANG in the next unit. You should be able to maintain the position with the head lifted for a count of ten with no fatigue before you proceed with the HEADSTAND HANG. Repeat the DOLPHIN two or three times. Massage your neck, shoulders and arms when finished. This pose is good following childbirth.

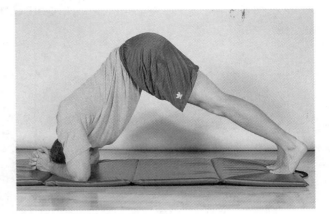

Figure 3.34A *Dolphin*

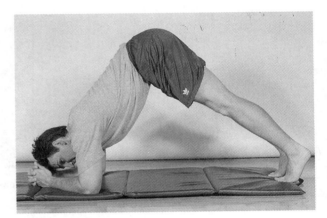

Figure 3.34B *Dolphin*

Moon Salute Routine

A popular form of practicing yoga is to do what are called "postural flows," or routines. This consists of doing a yoga pose and then moving smoothly to another pose using the breath to connect them. One of these, known as the MOON SALUTE, (Fig. 3.35) is a gentle stretching routine which moves the spine and improves the flexibility of the back. This routine is composed of the TRIANGLE (Fig. 3.29) and the TRIANGLE TWIST (Fig. 3.30). Remember to do the poses with all of the necessary corrections to achieve the correct alignment. This routine is a nice warm up and cool down stretching routine. Remember, for a smooth execution, the breath is the connector.

Moon Salute Routine

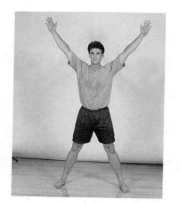

A. Reach to Sky: **Inhale.** Arms reach overhead

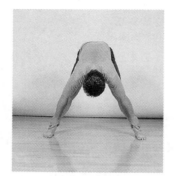

B. Bow to Earth: **Exhale.** Move forward from hips, lowering arms with hands on lower legs, head hanging down relaxing neck.

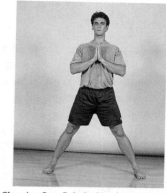

C. Shooting Star: **Inhale.** Hands together in front of chest, straightening arms & looking up.

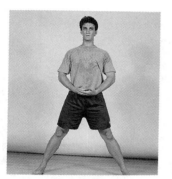

D. Full Moon: **Exhale.** Lower arms making a large circle until hands are together one on top of the other by lower abdomen.

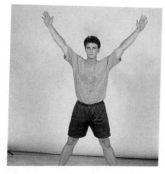

E. Pointed Star: **Inhale.** Raise arms out to side with palms down.

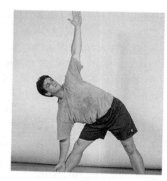

F. Triangle: **Exhale.** Go to the Left side, following direction for #29.

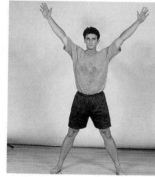

G. Pointed Star: **Inhale**

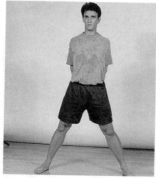

H. Shoulder Stretch: **Exhale.** Arms behind you allowing the neck & shoulder to relax.

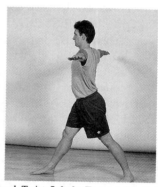

I. Trunk Twist: **Inhale.** Turn trunk to Left side.

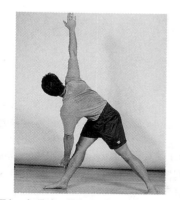

J. Triangle Twist: **Exhale.** On Left side follow directions for #30.

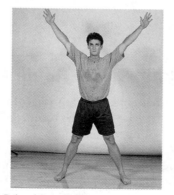

K. Pointed Star: **Inhale.**

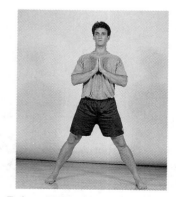

L. End pose NAMASTE: **Exhale.** Relax. Repeat to the Right side for F, I, and J.

Figure 3.35

BEGINNING YOGA PRACTICE SESSION

Do these routines whenever you want after you have learned the poses that are listed. Do each pose two-three times remembering to use your breath as it is taught when all of the basic instructions are presented. Always end with relaxation in the corpse pose.

Routine I	**Routine II**
Mountain Pose (Fig. 3.13)	Mountain Pose (Fig. 3.13)
Neck Stretch and Turn (Figs. 3.1 & 2)	Moon Salute (Fig.3.35)
Body Rolls (Fig.3.3)	Thigh Toner (Fig. 3.8)
Knee Thigh Stretch (Fig. 3.4)	Head of Cow (Fig. 3.19)
Cobra (Fig.3.14)	Chest Expansion (Fig. 3.20)
1/2 Locust (Fig. 3.15)	Cat (Fig. 3.21)
Fetus (Fig. 3.16)	Dog (Fig. 3.23)
Dog (Fig. 3.23)	Dolphin (Fig. 3.34)
Shoulder Stand (Fig. 3.25)	Shoulder Stand (Fig.3.25)
Fish (Fig. 3.26)	Fish (Fig. 3.26)
Tree (Fig. 3.28)	Abdominal Lift (Fig. 3.31)
Triangle (Fig. 3.29)	Triangle (Fig.3.29)
Back Push Up (Fig.3.32)	Triangle Twist (Fig. 3.30)
Sitting Forward Bend (Fig. 3.18)	Fetus (Fig. 3.16)
Feldenkrais Kneeovers (Fig. 3.10)	FeldenkraisKneeovers(Fig.3.10)
Relaxation (Fig. 6.1)	Relaxation (Fig. 6.1)

SUMMARY

This unit has the basic asanas. Refer back to this unit when you need to refresh your memory about one of these poses and the directions, the breathing patterns, benefits, precautions and recommendations. Everytime that you do the asanas you will want to incorporate these concepts:

> 1. Coordinate the breath to the asana
> 2. Be aware of what is being felt - the energy and the relaxation
> 3. Control the return to the starting position
> 4. Do a counter pose

Continue on to Unit 4, Intermediate Asanas. The next group of hatha yoga poses are best learned after you have learned these in this unit.   You may find some of the asanas in the next unit more difficult, or require more strength and flexibility to execute. Be patient with your self and your practice.

RESOURCES

Books

Dworkis, Sam. *ExTension*. New York, NY.: Poseidon Press. 1994.

Folan, Lilias. *Lilias, Yoga, & Your Life*. New York, N.Y.: Macmillan Publishing Co., Inc. 1981.

Iyengar, B.K.S. *Light on Yoga. New York*, N.Y.: Schocken Books, 1965

Smith, Bob. *Yoga For A New Age: A Modern Approach to Hatha Yoga*. Englewood Cliffs, New Jersey.: Prentice-Hall, Inc. 1982.

Videos

Lilias, Folan. *Lilias! Alive With Yoga. Vol. 1, 2 and 3*.

Walden, Patricia, *Yoga Journal's Yoga Practice for Beginners , Yoga Journal's Yoga Practice for Flexibility*, and *Yoga Journal's Yoga Practice for Relaxation* (with Rodney Yee). Healing Arts 321 Hampton Drive Suite 203y Venice, CA 90291. 800-722-7347

Yee, Rodney. *Yoga Journal's Yoga Practice for Strength*,   Healing Arts 321 Hampton Drive, Suite 203Y, Venice, CA 90201. 800-722-7347.

Equipment

Hugger Mugger Yoga Products, 31 W. Gregson Ave. Salt Lake City, UT 84115, 1-800-473-4888

"LiliPad."-yoga mat. Helen Esser PO Box 202 Clifton, VA 22024.

Living Arts, 2434 Main Street 2nd floor, Santa Monica, CA 90405. 1-800-2-living.

Body Bridge, by Arch/EEZ 1011 East Ginter Road, Tucson, AZ 85706 1-800-326-2724

YOGA PRO PRODUCTS BOX 7612 Ann Arbor, MI 48107. 1-800-488-8414

Yoga Mats PO Box 885044 San Francisco CA 94188. 800-720-yoga

Gravity Plus (Inversion Swing) P.O. Box 2182, La Jolla, Ca 02038 (619) 456-0926

ASANAS: Intermediate Hatha Yoga Poses

> *It's hard to grow up when we haven't grown in.*
> *I guess that's what growing up is-*
> *growing into ourselves.*
>
> . . . **Anne Wilson Schaef**

As you continue on with the poses described in this unit, please remember the suggestions discussed at the beginning of unit 3 . What makes doing yoga special is the combination of the use of the *awareness/concentration* on the alignment and the bodies response, the *breath,* and doing a *counterpose* to balance the body at the completion of an asana. As always, when doing hatha yoga allow yourself to be comfortable in the pose, but gently challenged. Read the precautions for each asana before progressing on to the execution.

ENJOY!

Lunge

Benefits: Improves the strength and flexibility of the legs, ankles and knees. Improves the flexibility of the hip flexors in the pelvis.

Precautions: Go slowly if there are old injuries to the knees or ankles.

Directions: Do this pose with the side to the mirror if possible. Start standing and then bend the knees and place the palms on the floor beside the feet, lining up the toes and fingers.Take the weight on the **right** foot and the hands as you place the **left** leg back with the toes on the floor and then let the **left** knee touch to the floor. There should be a stretch happening in the muscles of the thigh. Image that you are allowing the pelvis to sink toward the floor. The **right** foot should be directly under the knee so that a right angle is formed at the knee and ankle joint. If it is not there, move the foot forward or backward to get this right angle. Lift the **left** knee off the floor and raise the arms toward the ceiling. To end the pose place the hands back on floor next to the feet. Lift up, pivoting the feet. Repeat with the other leg with **left** leg forward and **right** leg back.

Breath: Breathe normally as you do the asana.

Recommendations: Make sure the right angle at the knee and ankle is maintained. Allow relaxation to take place to facilitate the stretch.

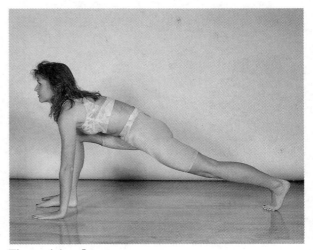

Figure 4.1   *Lunge*

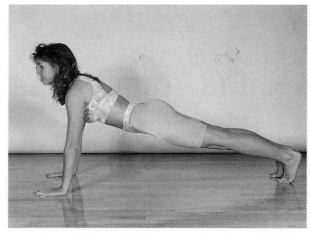

Figure 4.2   *Plank (Purvottasana)*

Plank (Purvottasana)

Benefits: Strengthens the muscles of the arms and shoulders.

Precautions: Make sure you do this pose in bare feet so that you don't slip. Be careful if you have old injuries to your arms or wrists.

Directions: Begin on all fours as in the CAT pose. Turn toes under and lift of the knees so that the body is straight like a board and weight is on the hands and toes. Rear end is down but back is not sagging. (similar to the up position in a push-up).

Breath: Inhale and then **exhale** as you lift of the knees. Breathe normally as you hold in the pose for about 6-10 seconds and then **exhale** as you lower the knees back to the floor.

Recommendations: Do this pose with your side to the mirror to check for straight alignment.

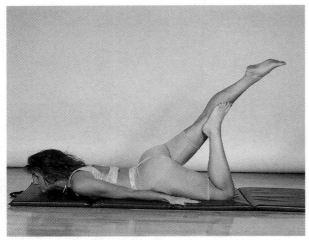

Figure 4.3   *Flying Locust*

Flying Locust

Benefits: Helps prepare the body for doing the full locust. Improves the strength and flexibility of the back. Strengthens the muscles of the buttocks and legs. Massages the uterus and intestines

Precautions: Do **NOT** do if you have injured the back, especially the lumbar area. Be gentle if you have had a problem with the sciatic nerve. Do **NOT** do when you are pregnant.

Directions: Lying on your abdomen with your chin on the mat, place the arms slightly under the body with the fists under the thighs. Bend your **left,** leg drawing the knee up. Contract the abdominal and gluteal muscles as you lift the straight **right** leg up and place it on the **left** foot. Relax, lower with control and repeat with bent leg.

Breath: Inhale and then lift the leg. **Exhale** as you relax. Breathing normal as you stay, and **exhale** as you lower.

Recommendations: It is important to keep the chin on the mat as that will keep the head straight and prevent muscle spasm in the neck. Extend the leg that is lifted, visualizing that you are lengthening it from the buttocks to the heel. Follow with the counterpose of the FETUS.

Full Locust (Salabhasana)

Benefits: Same as above but will strengthen the muscles of the back, buttocks, and legs more. Stimulates the circulation and the endocrine systems.

Precautions: Those with high blood pressure, injuries to the back, herniated discs in the lumbar area, heart ailments, or are pregnant should not do this pose.

Directions: Lying on your abdomen with chin on the mat. Place the fists and arms under the body so that the pelvis is resting on the arms. Gather your energy together, lift the muscles of the abdomen, tighten the muscles of the entire lower body, and LIFT both legs up. Keep the legs straight and stretch with toes pointed. Hold and then lower with control. Repeat 1-2 more times.

Breath: **Inhale** as you lift up, and **exhale** as you lower your legs. Take a deep breath before repeating.

Recommendations: Do not try to kick up, as the momentum will just bring you back down. You need to squeeze the buttocks together and LIFT. Practice daily to maintain back strength and to tone the leg muscles.

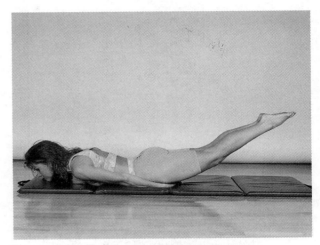

Figure 4.4   *Full Locust (Salabhasana)*

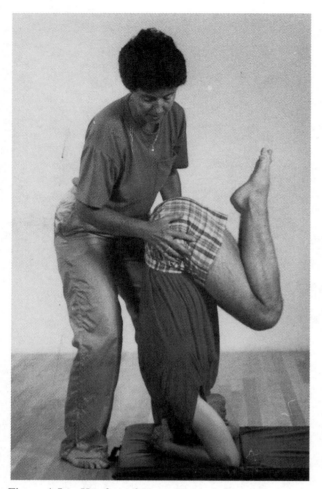

Figure 4.5   *Headstand Hang (Salamba Sirsasana)*

Headstand Hang (Salamba Sirsasana)

Benefits: This pose helps you gain confidence in your ability to balance your body in an inverted position without being afraid of falling. Again, the circulation is benefitted by this inverted position. Internal organs are allowed to move into a position where the weight of other organs had been shifted from them.

Precautions: This pose should not be done by those with high blood pressure, glaucoma, retina problems, thirty pounds overweight, a neck injury, head injury, brain surgery, or a hernia. Women are **NOT** to do this pose during their menstrual cycle or when pregnant.

Directions: This pose requires a partner who will "spot" you. You will kneel down in the position described for the DOLPHIN and the partner will stand behind your head with one foot by your hands and the other foot by one elbow. Their leg will be behind your back when you are in the pose and their hands on your hips to help you become stable. Lift into the DOLPHIN and then walk your feet in toward your body. When you are as close as you can be, then bend your knees bringing them to your chest and tilt the pelvis back slightly to find your center of balance. The partner can help by assisting with the lifting up and the centering of the pelvis. The hips will need to be back slightly toward their leg to counter balance the weight of the bent knees in the front. Partners do NOT let go, but as you feel them become more centered and balanced, you can lighten your touch until they can maintain the balance by themselves. Hold for twenty to thirty seconds. Lower down with control by bringing the feet to the floor first then lowering the knees. Keep your head on the mat while the partner massages your neck and shoulders. Lift up your head slowly so you don't get dizzy.

Recommendations: Practice this with a partner to spot you. Keep the shoulders lifted up from the ears. Do **NOT** slump down on to the neck. If you are having trouble with tilting the pelvis to find your center of balance practice pelvic tilts while lying on your back on the mat. Keep both elbows on the mat. Practice at this stage until you can easily maintain your balance without your partner holding you. For a counterpose do the CHEST EXPANSION.

Breath: The breath is very important as it helps you maintain a sense of control and stability. You make all your moves as you **exhale**.

1. **Inhale** - then **exhale** as you lift up to the DOLPHIN
2. **Inhale**- then exhale as you walk your feet in;
3. **Exhale** as you bring the knees to your chest and balance.
4. **Breathe** normally while in the HANG .
5. **Inhale** when you are ready to come down;
6. **Exhale** as you take your feet to the floor; **inhale**
7. **Exhale** as you lower your knees to the mat;
8. **Breathe** normally while you are being massaged. Doing the breathing in this manner assures your body of having the needed oxygen to do the pose.

Headstand (Sirsasana)

Benefits: All the benefits mentioned for the DOLPHIN and the HEADSTAND HANG are also gained from doing the HEADSTAND. In addition, you will improve your posture and gain self confidence.

Precautions: Do **NOT** do if you have a neck injury, hernia, glaucoma, retina problems, are overweight, or have high blood pressure. Women should **NOT** do during their menstrual cycle or when pregnant.

Directions: Begin by doing the DOLPHIN, then move to the HANG. While your partner is stabilizing you at your hips, straighten your legs. You will hold the pose for 20 seconds to two minutes. When you are ready to come down, do it slowly and with control, using your breath. You will bend your knees to the chest and then lower the toes to the mat ending in the DOLPHIN. Lowering the hips down, relax in the FETUS pose while the partner massages your back and shoulders.

Breath: The **inhale** is done and then the movement of straightening the legs is done as you **exhale**. Breath normally and full as you maintain the pose and then **exhale** as you lower the legs.

Recommendations: To maintain your balance, you need to contract the muscles of the quadriceps, and lengthen the muscles on the back of the thigh and calf. The abdominal and buttock muscles are contracted as this helps keep the lower back from arching. Keeping the elbows under the shoulders also helps prevent the back from arching. The head should be straight so that the weight will be centered on a spot on the top of the head. To help find this spot, put your index fingers on the top of your ears and move the fingers up until they meet on the top of the head. Bend down and place this area on the mat sliding the fingers away. When you are able to balance without the help of a spotter, practice by a wall or in a corner. As you become stronger you will be able to go up with the legs straight. Don't stay too long. Always retain some energy to control your coming out of the headstand.

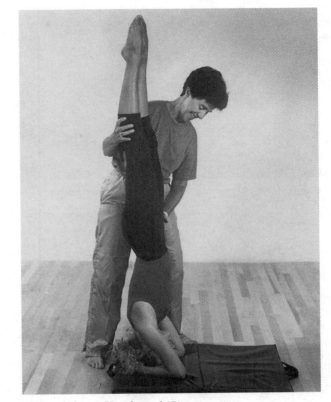

Figure 4.6A   *Headstand (Sirsasana)*

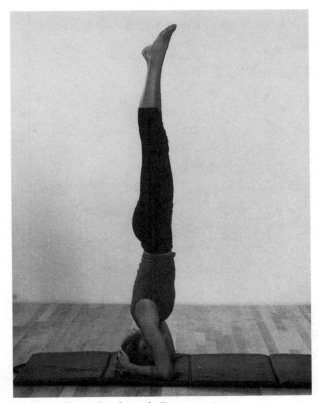

Figure 4.6B   *Headstand (Sirsasana)*

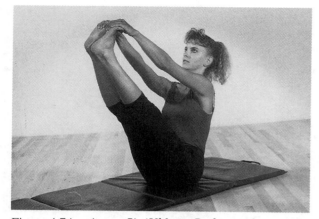

Figure 4.7A   *Arrow Sit (Ubhaya Padangusthasana)*

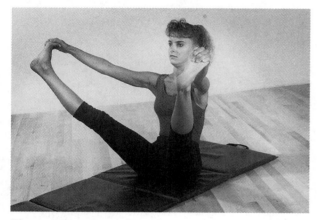

Figure 4.7B   *Arrow Sit (Ubhaya Padangusthasana)*

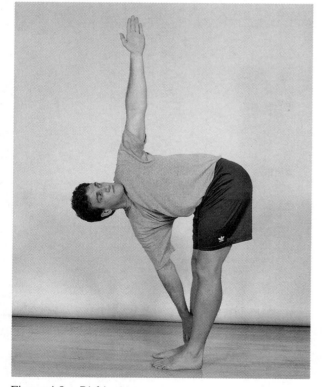

Figure 4.8   *Rishi*

Arrow Sit (Ubhaya Padangusthasana)

Benefits: Strengthens the abdominal muscles. Improves the flexibility in the legs.

Precautions: This pose will be uncomfortable for people who have injured their tailbones.

Directions: Sit with the knees bent and hands holding on to the toes. Lift the feet off the mat, tiltback and balance on your buttocks. Slowly straighten out your **right** leg and then your **left** leg. Balance and hold. When you have mastered the balance, separate the legs as far as you can comfortably and then move them back together.

Breath: Inhale and then **exhale** as you make the movements.

Recommendations: Always do this on a mat or a padded surface. Do not force the legs straight if the hamstrings are tight. Make sure there is nothing behind you that you could hit your head on as you may roll back.

Rishi

Benefits: This pose balances and equalizes the sides of the body. You can also see the effects that yoga poses have on the circulation system.

Precautions: Do not hold the pose very long if you have high blood pressure, or eye problems such as glaucoma or trouble with the retina.

Directions: Standing erect, lift the arms and turn slowly to the **left**. Separate the arms placing the **right** hand on the inside of the **right** thigh and **left** arm is out to the **left** side. Slowly bend forward sliding the **right** hand down the **right** leg, bringing the **left** arm back so the spine is doing a twist and the **left** hand points to the ceiling. Keep the weight centered evenly on both feet and the hips directly over the feet. Lift up and bring the hands to the front and then repeat going to the **right** side. Do 2 more times on each side.

Breath: Inhale as you turn to the side and **exhale** as you bend forward. Breathe normally while you are in the pose. **Inhale** as you lift up and **exhale** as the arms return to the front and lower.

Recommendations: This pose can stretch the hamstrings but if it is too intense bend the knees slightly.

Balance Posture (Natarajasana)

Benefits: Improves the balance, posture and stretches the leg that is lifted. It also strengthens the support leg.

Precautions: This pose may be a challenge for someone who has sprained their ankle or had a foot injury. Be careful if you have knee problems - use the necktie.

Directions: Standing erect bend the **left** leg and reach down to hold the **left** ankle or foot with the **left** hand. The **right** arm is by the ear. Lean back slightly and then come forward allowing the **left** leg and arm to open up. Reach with the **right** arm and be strong with the **righ** leg. With control move slowly back to your beginning position and lower the leg and arm Repeat on the other side.

Breath: Keep breathing full and deep as it helps maintain the balance.

Recommendations: Focus on something as that will help you balance. This is a good preparation pose for the CAMEL. If you are not able to reach back to the foot, put a necktie around the foot and while holding it in your hand raise the leg and move into the pose.

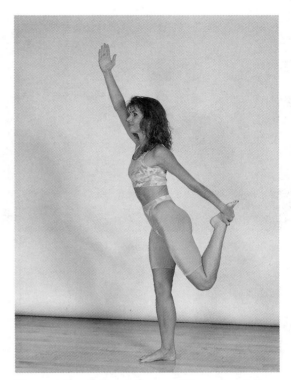

Figure 4.9   *Balance Posture (Natarajasana)*

Camel (Ustrasana)

Benefits: Improves the flexibility of the chest and spine. Strengthens the thighs and neck muscles.

Precautions: Be careful if you have problems with your neck or low back. If kneeling causes you pain, do not do this asana.

Directions: Do a CHEST EXPANSION and a BALANCE POSTURE as preparation poses. Kneel, pressing the shins down on the floor or mat and then do the CHEST EXPANSION bringing the hands down to hold the heels. Push the pelvis forward as this helps to keep the thighs perpendicular to the floor and over the knees. Lift the chest upward and allow the neck to stretch slightly, but do not drop the head back. Lift up out of the pose and continue moving forward and down into the FETUS pose for a counterpose.

Breath: Inhale as you do the CHEST EXPANSION. **Exhale** as you move into the position. Breathe normally as you hold.

Recommendations: Never do this without having done several preparation poses. Practice this facing a wall by bringing the thighs to touch the wall. Always do a counterpose to stretch the back.

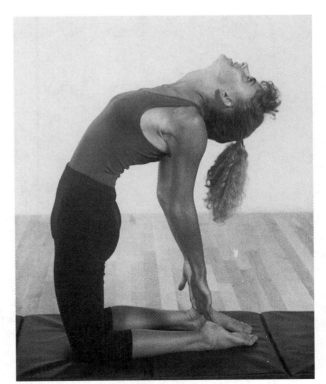

Figure 4.10   *Camel (Ustrasana)*

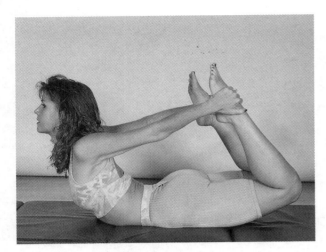

Figure 4.11   *Bow (Dhanurasana)*

Bow (Dhanurasana)

Benefits: Improves the flexibility of the back, shoulders and quadriceps. Strengthens the arms, and abdominal muscles. Massages the internal organs.

Precautions: Do not do if you have problems with the lower back or knees.

Directions: Lying on your abdomen, bend the knees and reach back to hold the ankles, or put a necktie around the ankles and hold the ends of the tie. With the thighs remaining on the mat, lift the chest. With the chest remaining on the mat, lift the legs so the thighs clear the mat. Now lift arms and legs from the mat. Arms are straight allowing the body to open up into the position. Hold, and if comfortable, slowly rock back and forth. Lower the chest and legs with control. Repeat when you are ready.

Breath: Inhale as you reach back to take the ankles and **exhale** as you lift up. You will probably breathe shallowly while on the abdomen.

Recommendations: Always do the FETUS pose as a counterpose.

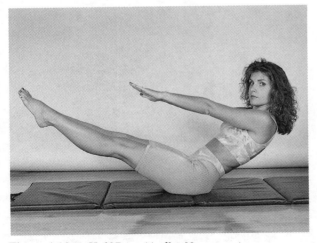

Figure 4.12   *Half Boat (Ardha Navasana)*

Half Boat (Ardha Navasana)

Benefits: Strengthens the abdominal muscles and the legs.

Precautions: This could be an uncomfortable position for someone with an injured tailbone. Be careful if you have lower back problems.

Directions: Sit erect with the knees bent and hands inter-locked behind the neck - but don't pull the head forward. Leaning back slightly, lift the feet from the floor and straighten the legs. Lower the legs until you are being challenged to maintain the pose and the abdominal muscles are strongly contracted and working. You can move the arms to make the pose more difficult- a) arms straight in front of you, b) arms out to the side, and c) arms up over the head. Bend the knees and lower the feet. Repeat.

Breath: Breathe normally as you do this pose. Do **NOT** hold the breath while you are holding the legs out.

Recommendations: Make sure you practice this on a padded surface. Do **NOT** do if you think it could bother your back .

Standing Straddle Forward Bend (Prasarita Padottonasana)

Benefits: Stretches and strengthens the legs, lengthens the spine, opens the hip joints, strengthens the arches of the feet, stretches the inner thigh and opens the shoulders. This pose also brings blood to the brain.

Precautions: Do not do if you have high blood pressure, glaucoma, or retina problems.

Directions: Place the feet 3-4 feet apart, and lifting the buttocks, fold forward while keeping the hips in line with the feet. Place the arms in 3 positions.

A. Place the hands on the folded arms allowing the weight of the arms to open the shoulders (10 seconds).

B. Straighten the arms and place the hands on the floor or blocks, directly under the shoulders. Bend the knees and lift the head stretching the chest forward-straighten the legs and allow the head to hang down.(10 seconds)

C. Place the hands on the lower legs and gently stretch the spine. Look up to help the scapula come toward the spine. Work in the pose for 10 seconds. To come up, release the arms to the side, round the back, bend the knees and start bringing the feet together by turning in the toes then, heels, then toes until the feet are together.

Breath: Inhale and then **exhale** as you bend forward and breath deeply as you relax into the positions.

Recommendations: Do this pose when the body has been warmed doing other asanas. Bending the knees will take the stretch of the legs and you can bring your awareness to the spine and shoulders and how they are stretching. Come up slowly.

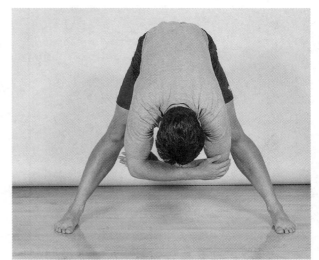

Figure 4.13A   *Standing Straddle Forward Bend (Prasarita Padottonasana)*

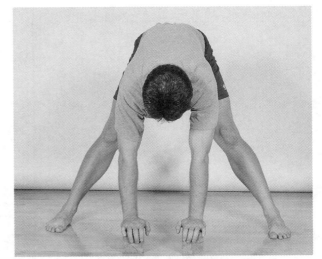

Figure 4.13B   *Standing Straddle Forward Bend (Prasarita Padottonasana)*

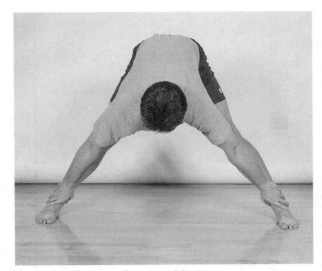

Figure 4.13C   *Standing Straddle Forward Bend (Prasarita Padottonasana)*

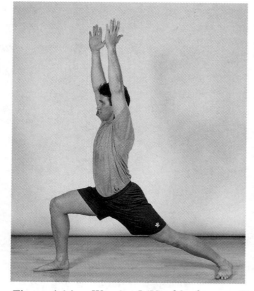

Figure 4.14   *Warrior I (Virabhadrasana I)*

Warrior I (Virabhadrasana I)

Benefits: This pose improves the flexibility and strength of the ankles, knees, hips, and shoulders. Balance and concentration also are enhanced. You gain a feeling of strength - like a warrior.

Precautions: It is important to monitor the knee and keep it facing the same direction as the toes. If you have had knee surgery this could be a challenge - but would eventually strengthen the knee.

Directions: With the legs apart 3-4 feet BOTH arms are raised over the head near the ears. Turn the **right** foot and torso to the **right** and bend the **right** knee until it forms a **right** angle over the ankle.   The **right** thigh should be parallel to the floor. The **left** foot is turned in slightly and the **left** leg remains straight with the muscles of the arch pulled up and the weight on the outer border of the foot. Visualize the upper body lifting up out of the pelvis and the pelvis area then sinking toward the floor. The focus is upward toward the hands with the head slightly back. Relax and work in the pose for a count of 10.   Straighten the legs, turn the feet to face the front, then pivot to the **left** and do the pose on that side.

Breath: Inhale, and as you exhale jump to the straddle position. Inhale as you lift the arms and torso up and **exhale** as the knee bends and torso turns toward the bent knee. Breathe normally while holding the pose and **inhale** as you lift up. **Exhale** and reflect before repeating to the other side.

Recommendations: If the bent leg is not able to have the thigh parallel to the floor, practice sitting in a straddle position with the thigh on a chair seat (Fig. 4.15B). In this partially supported position you are also able to make the corrections to the bent knee and also to the back leg and foot. It helps to remember the WARRIOR poses by counting the arms as viewed from the side. In this pose you see only one arm- they are as a pair.

Warrior II (Virabhadrasana II)

Benefits: They are the same as they are in WARRIOR I except that there is more strengthening of the shoulder muscles. This pose also improves posture in the shoulder area.

Precautions: Same as above. In addition, if there is an old shoulder or arm injury, this pose may bring it to your attention.

Directions: The leg position is identical to WARRIOR I. In this pose, the arms are extended out in a straight line from the shoulder with the palms down. The torso remains facing forward and the head turns to focus on the hand that is extended out beyond the bent knee. Straighten the leg, prepare the feet to repeat to the other side.

Breath: **Inhale** as you prepare and **exhale** as you jump into the straddle position. **Inhale** as you check the position of the torso and arms. **Exhale** as you bend the knee. Breathe freely and deeply as you hold the pose for 10-20 seconds.

Recommendations: Keep the spine upright and centered over the pelvis. Keep the shoulders rolled back and down from the ears. The arms are energized as you reach and extend from the shoulders, elbows, wrists and fingers. Monitor the bent knee to keep it over the heel - don't allow it to roll inward.

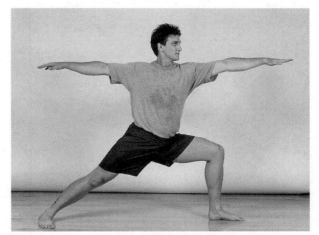

Figure 4.15A   *Warrior II (Virabhadrasana II)*

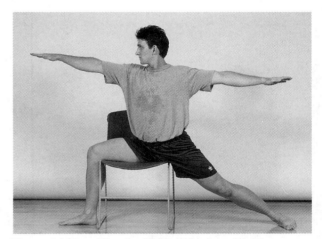

Figure 4.15B   *Warrior II (Virabhadrasana II)*

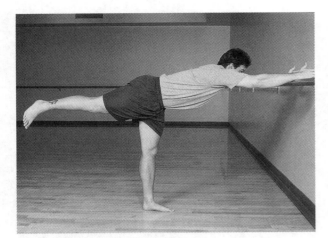

Figure 4.16   *Warrior III (Virabhadrasana III)*

Warrior III (Virabhadrasana III)

Benefits: This is a fun and challenging pose that greatly strengthens the legs and improves balance and concentration.

Precautions: The same precautions apply for WARRIOR III as are listed above. Balancing on one leg with the body leaning outward from the pelvis is more risky. If a person has balance problems, practice with the wrists on:
1. The extended arm of a partner
2. Back of a chair
3. The ballet barre

Directions: Go into Warrior I, lean out over the bent leg reaching forward with the hands. Be aware of a grounding of the heel. When you are at your maximun extension in this direction merely straighten your bent leg and the back leg will lift from the floor automatically. Your gaze is focused on the hands. It is very helpful to have a partner assist you in the correct alignment of the arms, trunk and extended leg and heel which are all in a straight line. The support leg should have the quadriceps contracted and the leg firm but not hyperextended at the knee. Hold in the pose 10 seconds . Lower with control and Repeat to the other side.

Breath: The breath is very important in the balance poses. Maintaining an even, deep breath keeps control of the asana. **Inhale**, and **exhale** as you go out into the straddle. **Inhale** and **exhale** into WARRIOR I, then **inhale** as you lower over the bent leg and **exhale** as you lift. Maintain a deep regular breath as you hold. When you are ready to end the pose **inhale** and then **exhale** as you bend the support leg and lower the other leg. **Inhale** up into WARRIOR I. **Exhale** as you lower the arms and face front.

Recommendations: The breath is a key ingredient in the execution of this asana as is the concentration of the focus. As the support leg becomes stronger you will also gain in your control. Practice with a partner . Do not allow the lumbar area of the spine to collapse. Use the abdominal muscles. Pat yourself on the back when you have successfully done this pose, alone and with control from start to finish!

Half Moon (Ardha Chandrasana)

Benefits: This pose also strengthens the legs, back shoulders and neck muscles. You gain in balance and concentration.

Precautions: Again, if a person has had problems with a knee or hip, this may be a challenge. An injury to a shoulder or arm may also cause some discomfort when making the final alignment corrections. Using a wooden block under the hand that is down will help with your stability in the pose. Don't hyperextend the knee of the support leg.

Directions: From TADASANA jump out with the feet 3-4 feet apart. Do the TRIANGLE and place the block about a foot in front of your support foot. Bend the knee of your support leg and place your hand on the block. Have the muscles of the back leg contracted and feeling strong. As you straighten your support leg your back leg will lift. The hips should be over the support leg with the top arm reaching up directly over the lower arm. The extended leg and trunk are in a line and are parallel to the floor. The arms and support leg should be perpendicular to the floor. Hold for 10 -20 seconds. Lower down to WARRIOR II by bending the support knee. Straighten the leg and jump back lightly to TADASANA. Pause and take a deep breath and repeat to the other side.

Breath: Inhale in TADASAN A and **exhale** as you jump out to the TRIANGLE. **Inhale** as you bend the knee, placing the hand on a block or floor. **Exhale** as you straighten the bent leg to lift into the pose. Breath steady and deep as you hold the asana and then **inhale** and **exhale** as you bend the knee and lower the leg following with an **inhale** while in WARRIOR II. **Exhale** as you jump back to TADASANA. Pause and take a deep breath before repeating.

Recommendations: Practice using the block - it takes greater control and flexibility to take the hand all the way to the floor. Don't sacrifice good alignment by trying to be "macho." Use your breath for energy to hold and to stay focused.

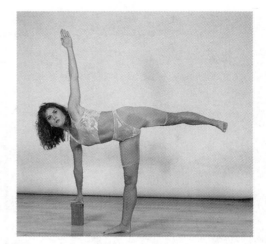

Figure 4.17   *Half Moon (Ardha Chandrasana)*

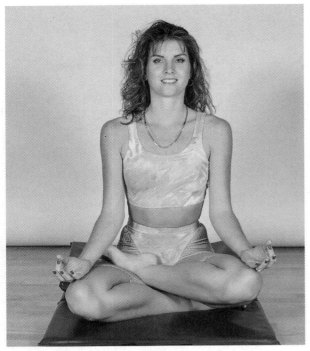

Figure 4.18A   *Half Lotus (Ardha Padmasana)*

Half Lotus (Ardha Padmasana) & Lotus (Padmasana)

Benefits: Learning to sit in these cross-legged positions brings about a feeling of stability and improves the flexibility of the joints of the legs and feet. These positions are recommended for meditation.

Precautions: If there has been an injury to the ankle, knee or hip, these positions may need to be adapted.

Directions:

Half Lotus. Begin by making sure that you are sitting with the weight evenly placed on both of the pelvis bones known as the ischium. The spine should be erect and the head directly over the spine. The legs are extended. Bending the **right** knee, pull in the foot until it is touching the body. The **left** leg is then bent and the **left** foot is placed on the top of the **right** thigh near the groin. Sit for awhile in this position and then change so the **right** foot is placed on the **left** thigh.

Lotus. You place each foot on top of the opposite thigh and as close to the groin as possible. You are able to see the sole of the foot.

Breath: This sitting position is ideal for the deep abdominal breathing and also for the Alternate Nostril breath (Unit 5.) Keep the breath full and deep and keep your awareness on your breath.

Recommendations: Do not be discouraged if you find this position very difficult. There are many factors that are involved - flexibility in the hips and pelvis, injury or surgery to the knee, how round or slim you are, and even the ratio of leg length to torso length. To assist with your adaptation to this pose, try elevating the pelvis on a folded blanket or a solid pillow. This opens the angle at the hips, is usually more comfortable, and also allows the spine to be in its natural alignment.

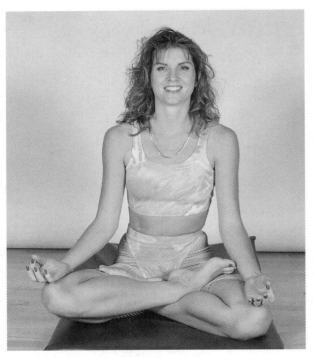

Figure 4.18B   *Lotus (Padmasana)*

Plough (Halasana)

Benefits: This pose is considered to be controversial because of the possible hyperflexion of the neck and strain on the ligaments between the pelvis and the spine. With adaptations any strain in those two areas can be prevented. It can provide a nice stretch for the back and the legs. It also stimulates the glands in the neck.

Precautions: Do with caution if you have injured your neck or have a problem in the lower back. Do NOT do if there is high blood pressure.

Directions: This pose is done with the head placed on the floor and the shoulders on the edge of the mat like the SHOULDERSTAND was taught. This prevents the hyperextension of the neck and allows the neck to maintain its natural curve. Lift up into a SHOULDERSTAND and lower both straight legs toward the bench, wall, or the mat depending upon how flexibile your hamstrings are. Placing the feet on the bench or wall takes some of the weight off the ligaments of the sacral area and does not over-stretch and weaken this area. Hold for 20 seconds. Lift back up to the SHOULDERSTAND and slowly lower down out of the SHOULDERSTAND. Follow with a FISH and CHEST EXPANSION as a counterpose.

Breath: Inhale and **exhale** as you lower the legs. Breathe normally while in the pose.

Recommendations: This pose should be done with caution and should not cause problems if done carefully and not held very long. Do not turn the head while in the PLOUGH.

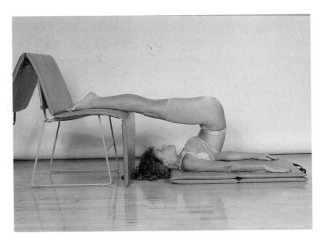

Figure 4.19   *Plough (Halasana)*

ROUTINES or "POSTURAL FLOWS"

There has been an interest in the 1980s and 1990s in putting a collection of yoga poses together to make a postural flow. There is the traditional approach as presented in the Salute to the Sun. There has also been a growing interest in the style of hatha yoga called Vinyasas. And quite recently there has been the Power Yoga or Ashtanga style being taught primarily in New York city and on the West coast. These developments will now be discussed with information about some of the leading teachers and samples of the various approaches.

Crocodile Routine

I learned the CROCODILE ROUTINE of Swami Dev Murti in England at the International Yoga Centre which he established. This routine is done on the floor on a mat and consists of variations of the spinal twisting pose of the crocodile. When the body is horizontal the spine is free and gravity is then affecting each vertebrae and muscular area evenly. The routine is very gentle and helpful for anyone with back problems so if this applies to you refer to unit 6 where it is presented in the section on Laughter (see Fig.6.4).

Salute to the Sun

One of the most popular routines which has appeared in many magazines for fitness enthusiasts is the SALUTE TO THE SUN (Fig. 4.20). The SALUTE TO THE SUN is a wonderful warm up routine that improves the flexibility of the spine and hips, and strengthes the arms. The whole body benefits from this routine. When you know the basic Sun Salute and can do it with all of the corrections and correct breathing pattern then move on to the 22 Step Version in the Power Yoga section.

Salute to the Sun (Surya Namaskar)

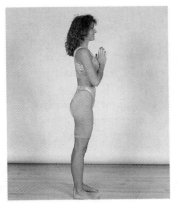

A. Tadasana: **Exhale**

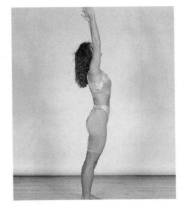

B. Slight Arch: **Inhale** *Tighten buttocks, lift rib cage & don't drop head back.*

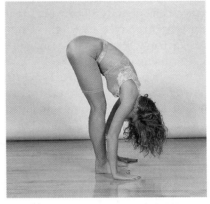

C. Standing Forward Bend. **Exhale.** *Place hands beside feet.*

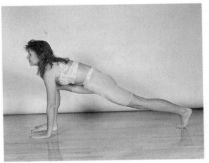

D. Lunge: **Inhale.** *Take Left foot back.*

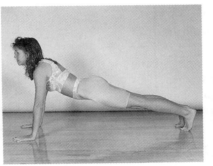

E. Plank: **Hold** *the breath.*

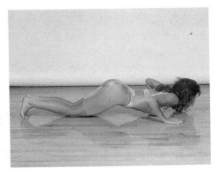

F. Knees & Chest: **Exhale.** *Lower the knees to mat, chest between the hands.*

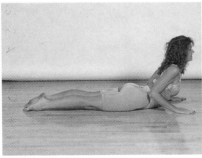

G. Cobra: **Inhale.**

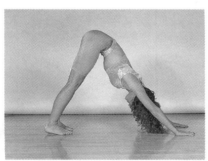

H. Dog: **Exhale.**

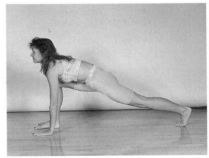

I. Lunge: **Inhale.** *Bring Right foot up between hands*

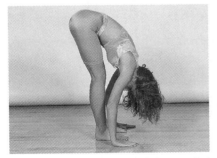

J. Standing Forward Bend: **Exhale.** *Bring Left Leg up.*

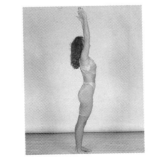

K. Slight Arch: **Inhale.** *Tighten buttocks and lift rib cage.*

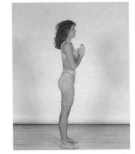

L. Namaste: **Exhale.** *Hands together.*

Figure 4.20

Repeat the routine again reversing the feet in the LUNGE.

Vinyasa

The "vinyasa" style of practicing yoga has grown considerably. The word means " to go step by step". This style of yoga is taught in India by Desikachar, whose father Krishnamacharya also taught B.K.S. Iyengar. Desikachar is recognized as one of the most important Yoga teachers in the world. He studied engineering and was an engineer for five years before returning to yoga teaching. He lives in Madras, India. Ian Rawlinson, an Englishman , who has studied extensively with Desikachar is one of the main teachers of this style in the United States.

There is a sequence of asanas that prepare you for a "goal" asana and then a series of asanas that are counterposes and allow a tapering down of the energy level and a balancing of the body. This approach is similar to the "3 Segment Workout" of Western exercise - looking at "Warm-up, Main Bout, and Cooldown." One of the most key factors, though, is the intense concentration and use of the breath in all of the postures and between the postures. The number of times a pose is done is counted by "how many breaths" - rather than repetitions of the movement. This contributes to the breath awareness and reminds the practioner that the breath is the source of the energy.

The breath also gauges the speed of the movement. The breathing instruction in this form of yoga has the breath move from the top to the bottom with the INHALE and from the bottom to top with the EXHALE. This is the reverse of what is usually taught and may require some extra practice time before coordinating it to the movement in an asana.Variations in the posture are recommended to modify the asana for individual differences. For example, when doing a standing forward bend, or a sitting forward bend if the stretch on the hamstrings is becoming too much by the last breath bending the knees slightly will lighten the hamstring stretch.

Another factor to consider is how you actually do the asana. Sometimes you have two choices or you can chose to do them both ways.
1. STATIC means you hold in the pose as you do your designated number of breaths.
2. DYNAMIC means that you move- you lift as you **Inhale** and you lower further as you **Exhale,** as you do your designated number of breaths. The style in which the Vinyasa are taught is with stick figure drawings. Following is the Shoulderstand-Vinyasa (Fig. 4. 21) that was an assignment in a workshop I attended with Ian Rawlinson.

SHOULDERSTAND - VINYASA

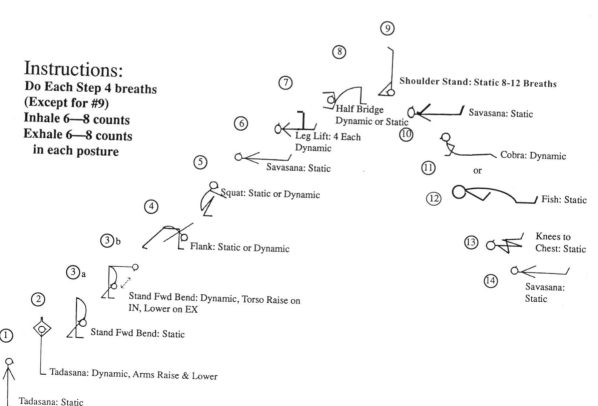

Figure 4.21 *Shoulderstand -Vinyasa*

PARTNER YOGA

Doing PARTNER YOGA is great fun and a wonderful learning experience in working with and valuing another human. A partner can assist you in your stretching. It is important that you and the partner are close to the same size and have a similar level of flexibility. You need to be gentle with each other; moving into the positions carefully. A sample partner yoga session follows in Fig. 4.22. Desiginate one of you Partner A and one of you Partner B and then follow the directions.

Partner Yoga

A. Knee-Thigh Stretch: Sitting erect with your backs touching "A" sits with the sole of the feet on the floor, knees bent and partner "B" has the soles of the feet touching and knees out to the side. Partner "A" reaches back and places the hands on partner "B's" thighs and gently exerts downward pressure until "B" says stop. Reverse positions.

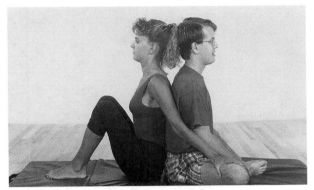
Figuree 4.22A   *Knee-Thigh Stretch*

B. Spinal Twist: Sit facing each other with legs crossed at ankles, backs erect and knees touching. Both place your **left** arm behind your back and with your **right** arm reach around your partners **right** side to join hands with your partners **left** hand. Keep heads and shoulders level. Turn you head to the **left** and gently pull on each other to twist more to the **left**. Slowly turn back to face each other. Repeat turning to the **right** with the **left** arms around the partners **left** side.

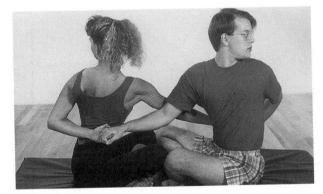
Figure 4.22B   *Spinal Twist*

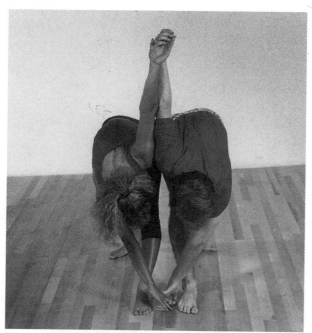

Figure 4.22C   *Windmill-Triangle Twist*

C. Windmill-Triangle Twist: Stand back to back, with your feet 3-4 feet apart and about 1 foot away from each other. Put the arms out to the sides with the hands lightly joined. Both turn to the SAME direction and pivot the heel of that foot to 90°. Lower the pair of arms on that side down and allow this pair of "inside" arms to continue moving down passing between the bodies until the joined hands move upwards to point to the ceiling. The "outside" arms with the hands pivoting inside of each other, have come down to the lower leg, ankle or floor depending upon the flexibility of the two of you. Reverse to come back up and repeat on the other side. Keep the legs straight and go slowly to enjoy the stretch through each phase.

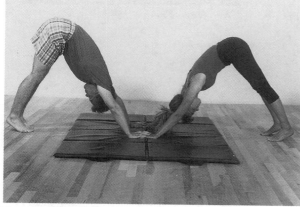

Figure 4.22D   *Dog*

D. Dog: Kneel down and sit back on your heels three feet away from each other, facing your partner. Place your extended arms on the mat and interlock your fingers with your partner's. Keep palms flat on the floor and shoulder distance apart. Sit back all the way on your heels, arms straight and forehead on the mat. Come up leaning to your **right** sides so that you are on your hands and knees. Turn your toes under, **inhale** and lift the buttocks up so you are in the DOG pose. **Exhale** and move into a full stretch while being anchored by your partners hands. Breathe and enjoy. Lower down and both relax in the FETUS pose.

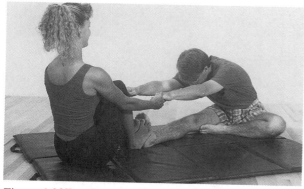

Figure 4.22E   *Partner Alternate Leg Stretch*

E. Partner Alternate Leg Stretch: Partner "A" sits with the **right** leg straight and the sole of **left** foot next to the inner **right** thigh. Partner "B" sits with the knees bent and the soles of the feet flexed against partners flexed **right** foot. Both **inhale**. Lift chests and clasp hands or wrists, arms straight. Partner "B" gently draws "A" slightly forward with a straight spine and **right** leg. Hold at "A's" comfortable stretch and release slowly. Change legs and repeat. Relax and then reverse position for "B" to be stretched in this pose.

F. Beam: Both kneel "thigh by thigh", with the outside leg out straight to the side, with toes pointing forward. Both raise arms and extend them upward. **Inhale** together and as you **exhale** lean to the outside with the outside arm lowered to rest hand on top of the lower leg. Inside arm follows the line of the trunk. Hold and breath normally. **Exhale**, as you lift up and reverse to repeat on the other side.

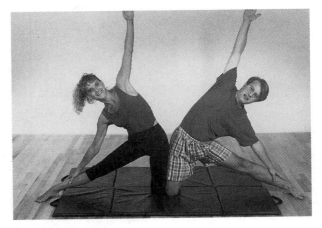

Figure 4.22F   *Beam*

G. Chest Expansion: This is a very "trusting pose". Stand facing your partner four feet away with your own feet three to four feet apart. Place hands on hips and keep the hips over the feet concaving the lower back as you lean forward leading with the chest. Place the hands palm to palm and straighten the arms up toward the ceiling. The foreheads touch and the buttocks are pushed backward. The closer and more straight the arms are the greater the stretch in the pectorals. Release the hands slowly, straighten up, and massage each others shoulders.

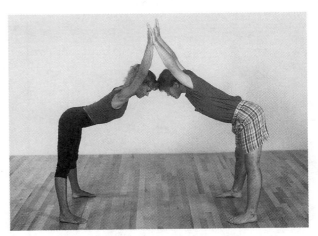

Figure 4.22G   *Chest Expansion*

H. Cobra: (Do NOT do if you have back problems). Partner "A" lies prone, clasps the hands behing the back as in the chest expansion position. Partner "B" kneels on each side of "A's" knees. Partner "A" lifts chest from floor as in the COBRA and then "B" takes "A's" clasped hands and *gently* brings her further into the pose. Hold and lower slowly and do the next pose before reversing positions.

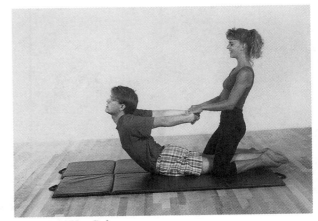

Figure 4.22H   *Cobra*

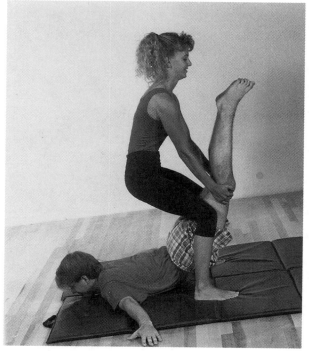

Figure 4.22I   *Locust*

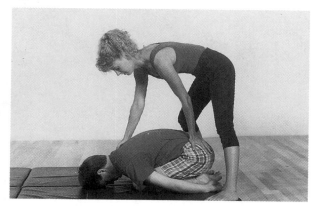

Figure 4.22J   *Massage*

I. Locust: (Do NOT do if you have back problems). Partner "A" lies prone with the hands on the floor by the thighs. Partner "B" stands by "A's" knees facing "A's" feet with her knees bent. Partner "A" lifts both legs and then "B" places hands under "A's" thighs and "B" straightens her legs to gently bring "A" into a higher position. Partner "B" should let the muscles of the thigh do the lifting NOT the back. "B" lower "A's" legs to the floor and then "A" rests in fetus pose while "B" massages "A's" back (Fig. 4.22J). Reverse and now do the COBRA and the LOCUST for partner "B".

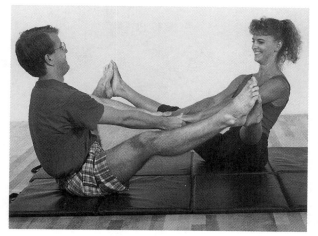

Figure 4.22K   *Partner Arrow Sit*

K. Partner Arrow Sit: Sit facing each other, knees bent, heels on floor and toes pushing against partners toes. Join hands on the outside of the legs. Backs are erect. Slowly straighten up one pair of legs and then the other. Now, without letting the feet and legs touch to the floor trade places with the arms so the legs are out in a wide "V" and the joined hands are now in the center. Lift the arms, bend the knees and return to the starting position. Repeat two more times.

ASHTANGA VINYASA YOGA (Power Yoga)

> *"Doing Power Yoga has made me*
> *Fitter and Stronger".*
> Sting, *Mens Health,* **May, 1995. p.93**

This is a form of yoga that is very ancient but was only rediscovered in the 1930s when a lost manuscript , *Yoga Kurunta,* was found in the archives of a Calcutta University by T. Krishnamacharya. His student, K. Pattabhi Jois, and collegeaus translated it from the Sanskrit and Jois began teaching it in Mysore, South India. He will be 80 years old in 1996 and is highly respected among his many students around the world. Two Americans traveled to India to study with Jois and were finally accepted as students. Since that beginning in the early 1970s and their return to the United States classes have been developing. In New York City at the New York Road Runners Club, Beryl Bender Birch and her husband Thom Birch have been teaching Power Yoga for fifteen years. The publication of her book of the same name is based on the program she has been teaching.

For more than twenty-five years, Bikram Choudhury has been teaching a challenging 90 minute workout at the Yoga College of India in Beverly Hills CA. An account of having participated in sixteen of these classes was written by a 49 year old male, and was published in the *U.S. News and World Report*, (May 16 1994). Mike Tharp had this to say of his experience ". . . I already see results. Although, I am years from being even close to competence, I'm more flexible, I concentrate better. I sleep more soundly, my appetite is more moderate, my sex life is sexier. My breathing had deepened so much that I can now hit the high notes in 'Crying' along with Roy Orbison" (p.83).

There are some characteristics of Ashtanga yoga that make it different from other approaches of Hatha Yoga. There are three techniques combined together:

> 1. **UJJAYI** breathing (taught in unit 5)
> 2. **UDDIYANA BANDHA** which is done when the abdominal lift is practiced
> 3. **MULA BANDHA** which is a contraction of the pelvic floor muscles including the anal sphincter and the vaginal muscles.

When all three of these techniques are added to the execution of the yoga poses there is a building of inner heat and this is what is one of the attractions of doing this style of yoga. Another aspect of doing Ashtanga yoga involves directing your gaze to assist you in staying focused and in control of the asana. Doing Ashtanga yoga is a more advanced approach and is recommended only after the correct alignment and breathing has been accomplished in all of the asanas. The poses and bandhas are held for five breaths.

In 1993 Richard Freeman from Boulder, CO, made a two hour video tape, *"Yoga with Richard Freeman,* Ashtanga Yoga The Primary Series." A 96 page handbook with photos and directions accompanies this video. This video is beyond the begining level and is challenging but wonderful to work with. See the resources at the end of this chapter for ordering information.

Learning the 22 Step Variation of the Sun Salute is a start toward doing Power Yoga. On page 70 is a POWER YOGA ROUTINE that you should practice for a few weeks before doing one of the commercial videos.

22 Step Variation of Sun Salute

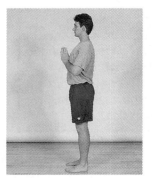

1. Beginning Pose: **Exhale.**

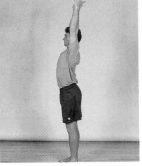

2. Slight Arch: **Inhale.** *Tighten buttocks, lift rig cage & don't drop head back.*

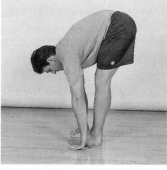

3. Standing Forward Bend. **Exhale.** *Place hands beside feet.* **Inhale.** *Take Left foot back to Lunge.*

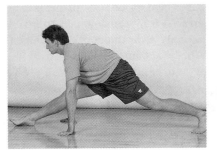

4. Standing Hamstring: **Exhale.** *Straighten front leg (right)* **Inhale** *- go to Lunge*

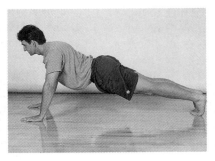

5. Plank: **Hold** *the breath*

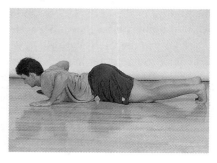

6. Knees & Chest: **Exhale.** *Lower the knees to mat, chest between hands.*

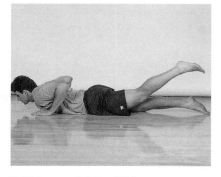

7. 1/2 Locust: **Inhale.** *Lift Leg.* **Exhale**. *Lower - Repeat other leg*

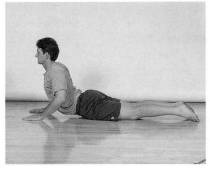

8. Cobra: **Inhale.**

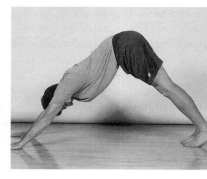

9. **Dog: Exhale.**

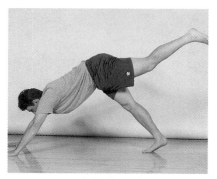

10. Lift L leg up behind as **Inhale**

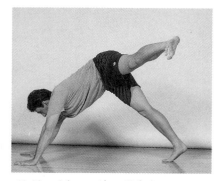

11. Move L leg to side as **Exhale**

Figure 4.23

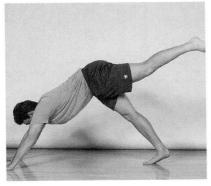

*12. Move L leg up behind: **Inhale.** Lower as **Exhale** and bring R. foot up to Lunge*

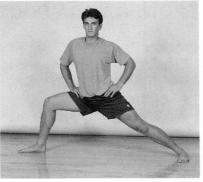

*13. Lunge with Spinal Twist: R Hand on R knee, **Inhale** as L hand on L hip turn to L. **Exhale** to front*

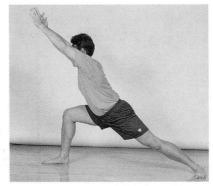

*14. Arm Stretch Forward: **Inhale** reaching out with back straight.*

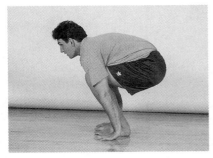

*15. To Squat: L leg forward and hands to floor as **Exhale.** **Inhale:** straighten legs.*

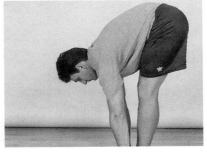

16. Standing Forward Bend

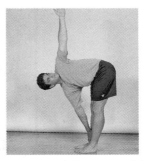

*17. Rishi: **Inhale** turning to L. **Exhale** Straighten and arms come to front.*

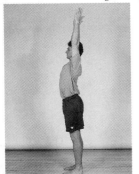

*18. Slight Arch: **Inhale.** Tighten buttocks & lift rib cage*

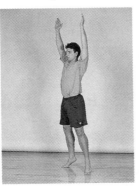

*19. Balance on Toes: **Exhale - Inhale** into pose turning L.*

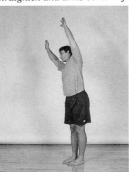

*20. Side Sway: **Inhale** as lean to R. **Exhale** center. **Inhale** to L. **Exhale** center.*

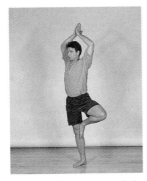

*21. Tree: L. leg up on **Inhale**. **Exhale** lower.*

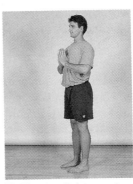

22. Namaste: Palms together.

Repeat the routine again reversing the legs in the Lunge and in 10, 11,12 and 21.

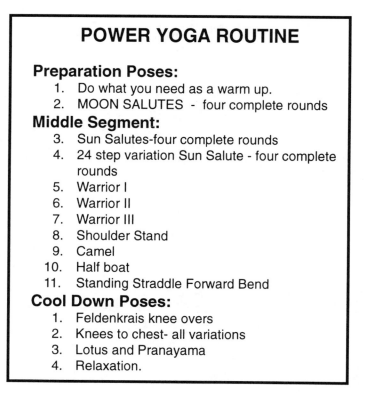

POWER YOGA ROUTINE

Preparation Poses:
1. Do what you need as a warm up.
2. MOON SALUTES - four complete rounds

Middle Segment:
3. Sun Salutes-four complete rounds
4. 24 step variation Sun Salute - four complete rounds
5. Warrior I
6. Warrior II
7. Warrior III
8. Shoulder Stand
9. Camel
10. Half boat
11. Standing Straddle Forward Bend

Cool Down Poses:
1. Feldenkrais knee overs
2. Knees to chest- all variations
3. Lotus and Pranayama
4. Relaxation.

INTERMEDIATE LEVEL TEACHERS

Iyengar Classes

The Iyengar certified teachers are all trained to offer intermediate and advance level classes. The address of the Iyengar Institute can be found in the resource section.

Ganga White and Tracy Rich

This delightful couple own the "White Lotus Foundation" in Santa Barbara, CA where they conduct classes and also teacher training workshops and retreats. Their video is also a challenging workout and their delightful personalities and calm centeredness as they instruct contributes to an enjoyable yoga session (see Resources).

Kalli Ray

Kalli Ray owns the Tri Yoga Center in Santa Cruz, CA, and also has an enjoyable video tape with the background music composed by her musician/husband, Mercury Max. She conducts daily classes, seminars and retreats. Kalli Ray's style of yoga is flowing and dance-like and her voice is soothing as it gives the directional cues. There is a strong emphasis on the breath as you are instructed in the Kriya Flows. This is an excellent tape for at home practice (see resources).

RESOURCES

Books

Birch, Beryl Bender. *Power Yoga: The Total Strength and Flexibility Workout.* New York, N.Y.: A Fireside Book, Simon & Shuster. 1995.

Dworkis, Sam. *ExTension.* New York, N.Y. : Poseidon Press. 1994.

Rawlinson, Ian. *Yoga for The West: A Manual for Designing Your Own Practice.* Sebastopol, CA P.O. Box 1460. 95473. CRCS Publishing

Publications

Cushman, Anne. "Kali Rays Tri Yoga". *Yoga Journal.* March-April. p. 58-65.

Eller, D. "The New Yoga." *American Health.* V12, July/August, 1993. p. 58-63.

Kilmurray, Arthur. "Yoga for Hips & Thighs". *Yoga Journal.* May /June. 1989. p. 60-69, 98-100.

Moyer, Donald. "Ardha Chandrasana- Half-Moon Pose". *Yoga Journal,* Nov/Dec/ 1992. p.42-44, 46,48-50.

Rawlinson, Ian. "Breathing and Vinyasa". *Yoga Journal.* Jan-Feb. 1988. p, 54-59.

_____ "Vinyasa and Counterpose". *Yoga Journal.* November/ December. 1986. p. 46-52.

Whitwell, Mark. "The Life and Yoga of Krishnamacharya: An Interview with .TK.V. Desikachar." *Yoga Journal.* October, 1995. p.90-96, 139-140.

Organizations

Iyengar Yoga Institute of San Francisco. 2404 27th Avenue, San Francisco, CA 94116

Videos

Freeman, Richard. *Yoga with Richard Freeman,* Delphi Productions LTD, 3160 4th St., Boulder, CO 80304. (303) 443-2109

Ray, Kalli *Tri Yoga,* P.O. Box 7827, Santa Cruz, CA 95061 (498)464-8100

White, Ganga and Tracy Rich. *Aerobic Yoga* and *Total Yoga.* White Lotus Foundation, 2500 San Marcos Pass, Santa Barbara, CA 93105 (805) 964-1944

Pranayama: Breathing Techniques

> *Just as a child overcomes his clumsiness*
> *by becoming aware of his body and learning to walk,*
> *so does breath awareness gradually free the mind*
> *from relating to the breath on an unconscious level*
> *and this brings it under greater conscious control.*
>
> **. . . John Clark- Foreward to *Science of Breath***

WHAT IS PRANAYAMA?

This aspect of yoga addresses the flow of energy, lifeforce, or "Prana," through the body. "PRANA" means energy and "AYAMA" means expansion. Pranayama is not only the breathing exercises. The asanas have freed the body and thus the flow of prana throughout the body is enhanced. The prana, through the breathing patterns, connects to the use of the life force within the physical body. In pranayama there is a conscious attempt to use the nose, throat, lungs, diaphragm, abdominal and intercostal muscles of the ribcage to direct the prana. Many times when we experience tension, sorrow or anger, we instinctively first HOLD the breath and then take a deep breath to calm ourselves or to gather more energy to see ourself through a difficult moment. In yoga, the practice of pranayama is done with a conscious plan and is not left to instinct alone. Remember how the breath was a part of the execution of the asanas as they were taught in units 3 and 4? In this unit the benefits and techniques of the complete breath, Ujjayi breath, the alternate nostril, the Ha Breath with the abdominal lift, the Kapalabhati breath, and Bhastrika, the bellows breath, will be discussed. What research has discovered about the breath and recommendations for practice will also be presented.

Benefits

The following benefits are common to all of the types of yoga breath. The practioner learns to utilize the entire lung rather than only the upper portion which is the usual breath pattern. Also, the muscles used in breathing are strengthened and the elasticity of the ribcage is maintained. Respiratory problems such as asthma, allergies, sinus or nasal congestion can be helped by practicing these breathing techniques. They are also recommended for coping with stress and to calm, as well as energize, the body. Becoming aware of the breath and learning to control it leads to more respect for the importance of the respiratory system and how oxygen is needed by every cell in the body. This new awareness and concern for the health of their lungs has led some smokers to quit. Those in music and theater enjoy using these breathing techniques to enhance their control and ultimately their performance. Athletes and dancers also learn to value the breath control learned doing yoga.

I will mention a personal testimony to the power of pranayama and how it can come to your aid in a traumatic moment. When hurrying to prepare for an evening class, I slipped and fell, landing on my left elbow and smashing an armful of books, folders and video tapes into my left rib cage. My first response was one of having "lost" my breath and a pain in my ribs. Then the pain in my left elbow started. I had heard a sound and was pretty certain that I had broken something. I asked the people who saw me fall to get the athletic trainer to help me. I then noticed that I was very hot, thirsty, was breathing shallowly, and getting dizzy. I did not want to faint and fall on my arm again and I then realized that I was going into shock. So I told the bystanders " Don't be alarmed- I am not hyperventilating- I am doing my yoga deep breathing to calm my body. " I closed my eyes did a few rounds of the deep breath while sitting there on the floor. It was absolutely amazing how my body was retrieved from a state of shock - all of the symptoms mentioned were gone. I was informed that I had turned as green as my dress. I was then able to joke with them and said "Well, that is rather fitting - considering Green is my maiden name." Even in the midst of having broken the end of the elbow completely off, I was pleased to discover how my yoga training and my body's response came to my aid. It has continued to do so during the repair, recuperation and now rehabilitation. I don't recommend this "discovery method" for anyone else. Just take my word for it that the following breathing practices are well worth learning and practicing.

RECOMMENDATIONS

How to position yourself? First of all be, comfortable. Loosen your clothing so there is nothing tight around your waist. You can sit in a chair or on the floor with the legs crossed in whatever position is the most comfortable for you. Try sitting with the pelvis slightly elevated (3-6 inches) as the back can now stay more erect and the hip joints and legs are more relaxed. Some of the breathing techniques will be done lying and some standing.

When to practice the breaths? This will vary with the type of breath you are wanting to do. When you awaken in the morning and before you get out of bed and again at night are good times to do the complete breath as you already are in the correct position. Whenever you are feeling sluggish or tired during the day, take some breaths to perk yourself up. When you need calming down use the breath to help you. Refer to the diagram below (Fig. 5.1) of the respiratory system to familarize yourself with the area involved before you practice the following breathing techniques.

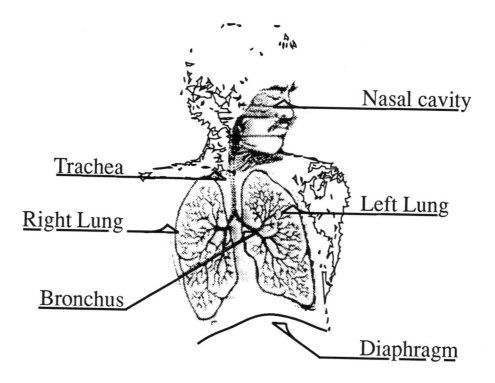

Figure 5.1 *Respiratory System*

> *To our ordinary consciousness,*
> *breathing only serves to maintain our body.*
> *But if we go beyond our mind,*
> *breathing can open up a completely new foundation for our life.*
>
> . . . **Illse Middendorf**

VARIETIES OF YOGA BREATHING

Complete Breath with *UJJAYI*

Technique: Position yourself in SAVASANA (the corpse pose in Unit 6). The **exhale** begins with the diaphragm moving upward slightly to begin pushing the old air out. At the end of the exhale, the abdominal and intercostal muscles will contract strongly. The abdomen will flatten and will continue to do so to empty the lung. The lower ribcage will squeeze inward.

To add to your control, you can use the throat muscles to assist you. Instead of "sniffing" the air in at the nose, draw it in at the throat. The glottis partially blocks the throat, slowing down the outgoing air. When this is done correctly you will here a sound similar to a "small wheeze." You also use the throat muscles to help control your exhalation and again there will be a sound. Once you have learned this technique, use it for your breath that is done when you are doing the asanas. You will maintain your energy for the execution of the asana. Place your hands on the abdomen to monitor the lifting upwards of this area on the first phase of your breath, then move your hands so you can feel the ribs to monitor their movement outward as this part of the lungs begin to fill, and finally, place your hands on the clavicles to monitor the upper part of the lungs filling. When you first begin to learn this breath, the movements may be slight but don't be discouraged. With practice your body will follow your mental commands to breathe in this fashion and eventually it will become a natural way for you to take a deep breath. When you exhale, let your hands follow the same areas as they return to their positions to end the complete breath.

Recommendations:

1. Practice this breath several times daily and you will be calmer
2. Do not practice on a full stomach
3. Do at night as it aids you in falling asleep
4. Begin with a count of six for your inhale and six for your exhale. Work up to doing the breath for five minutes and gradually increase your time to fifteen minutes. Following your breathing stay in SAVASANA for at least ten minutes

5. Practice the breath lying on your abdomen as well so you can be more aware of the breath as the body is expanding and pressing downward at the abdomen and chest area
6. For a consistent pranayama practice sit with the spine erect in one of the cross legged sitting asanas (HALF-LOTUS or LOTUS)
7. Maintain your concentration on the pass of the air through the nostrils and the sound it makes as it passes by the glottis
8. Also, it is very exciting to do the breath sitting back to back with a partner with the eyes closed. One does the complete breath and the other notices the feeling of the breath as it flows up and down their spine. This should be done after you both have been doing the breath for several weeks. This is very special as you are put in touch with this human in a way that is new to you both. You are "feeling" the life force within them and also noticing how the breath takes place in the back.

Ha Breath with Abdominal Lift

The basic instructions for this pose were presented in Unit 3 (p. 38) Practicing this breath brings you more in touch with your breathing muscles and strengthens them. This breath also prepares you to learn the KAPALABHATI and the BHASTRIKA breaths.

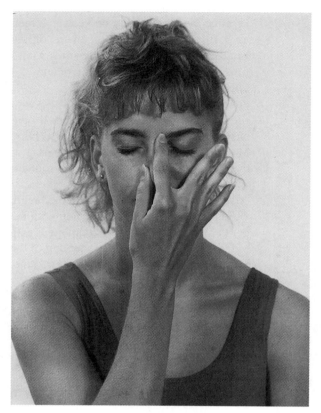

Figure 5.2   *Alternate Nostril Breath (NADI SHADHANAM)*

Alternate Nostril Breath (NADI SHADHANAM)

This PRANAYAMA practice involves inhaling through one nostril, then exhaling through the other; then inhaling on that side and exhaling through the nostril where you began (Fig. 5.2). The practice of this breath will bring about a balanced state. Just as the term " HA" refers to the sun it also refers to the right nostril. And consequently the term " THA" refers to the moon and the left nostril.

Technique: To begin, you should be sitting with eyes closed, spine erect, and head centered and level. Place your index finger on the bridge of your nose, with the thumb controlling the opening and closing of one nostril and the middle and ring finger controlling the other nostril. First, check the flow of air in each nostril , and begin the inhalation on the side that is most open. Inhale to a count of 4, 6, or 8 (whichever is most comfortable for your lung capacity), and exhale on the same count but through the other nostril. Then complete the round by inhaling on that side and exhaling on the side where you began. Repeat this cycle for a total of six times. Then take a normal deep breath and lie back or sit quietly to enjoy the calm feeling you have created for yourself.

There has been considerable research concerning the connection between the breath and the brain. The yoga belief has been that the breath needs to occur in both nostrils to keep the body in balance. It has been discovered that the brains electrical activity can be stimulated in one hemisphere or the other depending on which nostril the breath is concentrated. The breath in the right nostril activates the left hemisphere and the breath in the left nostril activates the right hemisphere as measured with an encephalogram. The autonomic nervous system and the hypothalamus have also been the subject of research using the breath (see *American Health*, November 1986, p.16 &18). The exact connection between the nose and the mind is not clear at this point, but hopefully science will find some answers to confirm what yogis have been doing for centuries.

YOGA NASAL CLEANSING PROCESS: NETI

This is a fitting place to discuss this yoga practice. Having been a person bothered with nasal/sinus congestion since childhood I was most happy to learn this yoga technique over 20 years ago. I am mentioning it here as society and the medical profession are now recommending the use of a salt water nasal wash to relieve congestion. This is a safe and ancient practice. Many people have been taught as children to gargle with warm salt water for sore throats. This nasal wash is a similar practice except that warm salt water is poured in one nostril at a time. It then drains out the other nostril, down the back of the throat, and some may dribble down your face. You then repeat the process on the other nostril (Fig. 5.2). The salt will shrink the swollen nasal membranes and the warm water will be soothing and flush away the congestion and dried mucus. This practice has been prescribed by ear, nose and throat physicians and now the pharmaceutical companies are making a saline water nasal douche that comes in a small plastic squeeze bottle. If you are bothered by chronic nasal problems share this technique with your physican for her/his input and refer to Table 5.1. for directions.

Directions for Water NETI

1. Dissolve 1/4 to 1/2 teaspoon sea salt in 1 cup of warm water. Use a measuring cup, tea pot or Neti pot shown in Fig. 5.2
2. Lean over a sink and tilt the head sideways to the **right** and place the spout of the pot into the **left** nostril. Pour in 1/2 of the salt water
3. Now tilt the head to the **left** and pour the remainder into the **right** nostril
4. Dry the nostrils and the back of the throat by doing the following
   a. tilt the head forward so the water may run out
   b. bend forward at the waist and exhale with force through both nostrils
   c. turn the head to the **right** and exhale with force
   d. turn the head to the **left** and exhale with force
   e. lift the head and inhale and immediately exhale through both nostrils
   f. repeat the procedures until the nostrils are dry

Table 5.1

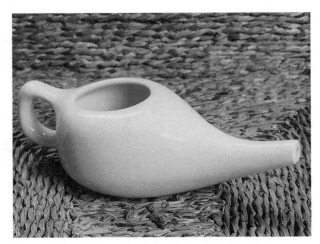

Figure 5.2 *Photo is used with permission of the Himilayan Publishers, RR1, Box 407, Honesdale, PA 18431.*

As reported in *Yoga International Reprint Series- Inner Body Cleansing: The Nasal Wash,* the medical textbooks researched by Fadal, in 1988, enumerated the benefits of the warm saline irrigations as follows:

---

1. Augments mucociliary flow
2. Liquefies tenacious mucus
3. Soothes irritated tissue
4. Removes crusts and microforeign bodies
5. Augments tissue repair
6. Reduces forceful nose blowing
7. Improves olfaction (sense of smell)

Kapalabhati

The Sanskrit word KAPALA means "skull" (which is similar to the Latin for head- *caput*), and BHATI means to make "clean." Thus, the meaning is literally "cleaning the skull." The nostrils, ears and the other air passages inside the head will be affected with this technique.

Technique: The breath can be practiced in a sitting po- sition with the spine erect and the head balanced. This breath involves a long, slow, passive inhala- tion and a rapid, forceful exhalation that contracts the diaphragm and abdominal muscles in order to empty the lungs. The shoulders do not move. On the exhalation, the air can be directed out the nos- trils similar to blowing your nose (you can hold a handkerchief under your nose). Repeat six more breaths, allowing the inhalation to just happen but working on the exhalation.   Begin with seven breaths and gradually work up until you are doing twenty-one.

Benefits: The benefits of KAPALABHATI   are numerous. This breath helps clear the sinus passages while stimulating the internal organs and toning the abdominal muscles. With the strong exhalation, the carbon dioxide level in the blood falls. Continuing the breath for two - three minutes cleanses the body and allows the cells to eliminate the carbon dioxide they produce. The normal level automatically returns soon after stopping. The cells become saturated with oxygen when they lose the carbon dioxide. Thus, this practice is working at the cellular level, and increases the ozygenation of the blood. The brain also benefits from this higher oxygen intake as the body is not demanding oxygen for muscular movement when sitting in a cross- legged position.   With regular practice of Kapalabhati the powers of concentration and memory are enhanced.

Precautions: It is not recommended for anyone suffer- ing from a lung condition. Those with heart dis- ease need a long preparation time with the other breathing techniques and need to have developed control of the abdominal muscles.

Bellows Breath (BHASTRIKA)

When doing this breath, the abdominal area will function like a bellows that expands and contracts. This is a more powerful breath and should be learned after KAPALABHATI has become an easy, natural breath to perform.

Technique: Sit in one of the crosslegged positions with the spine erect. The inhalation and exhalation are both vigorous and forceful and one immediately follows the other. It is done more quickly than the other breaths and the speed of the breathing gradually accelerates. Do not sacrifice a complete inhalation to the sake of speed. Again, there is a slight tightening of the glottis as in UJJAYI breathing.   Begin with a total of seven breaths gradually increasing until you are doing twenty-one.

This breath also clears the nasal passages and sinuses and stimulates the entire abdominal area. As in KAPALABHATI, respiration has been accelerated at the   cellular level thus bringing about a revitalisation.   This breath is not recommended for smokers as it may draw the residue of nicotine and tar deeper into the lungs. Do not do this breath if you are pregnant, have high blood pressure, heart disease or emphysema.

YOGA BREATHING FOR ASTHMATICS & OTHER LUNG CONDITIONS

The practice of the above mentioned yoga breathing techniques enable a person to develop a greater respect for their respiratory system. As a re- sult they then want to do what they can to enhance their use of the breath to assist their lungs in becom- ing more healthy. This will be discussed in greater detail in Unit 9, "Therapeputic Use of Yoga."

SUMMARY

These breathing techniques are tried and proven over centuries of practice by the yogis. It is well worth your time to practice them on your own to achieve the benefits that they have to offer you. These benefits range from calming you, to stimulating you, and to increasing your circulation. Refer to the resource listing for additional information.

> *Breathing in, I calm my body.*
> *Breathing out, I smile.*
> *Dwelling in the present moment*
> *I know this is a wonderful moment.*
> **. . . Thich Nhat Hanh from** *Being Peace.* **1988**

RESOURCES

Publications

"In One Nostril, Out the Other,"*Brain/Mind Bulletin,* August 1989.

Funderburk, James. Ph.D. *Science Studies Yoga: A Review of Physiological Data.*   Honesdale, PA. Himalayan International Institute of Yoga Science and Philosophy, 1977.

Farhi, Donna. " Moving with the Breath," *Yoga Journal.* Nov/Dec. 1992. p.77-83.

Hanh, Thich Nhat. *Being Peace.* Berkeley, CA:. Parallax Press. 1988

Hendricks, Gay. Ph. D. *Conscious Breathing.*   New York, NY: Bantam Books, 1995.

Iyengar, B.K.S. *Light on Pranayama.* New York, Crossroad, 1985

Laurence, Leslie. "Air Power," *Self,* May, 1991. p. 160-161, 186 &190.

Miller, Richard. "Working with the Breath," *Yoga Journal,* September/October 1989. P. 67-75.

_____   "The Breath of Life," *Yoga Journal,* May/June 1994. p. 82-90,140-142.

Rama, Swami. Rudolph Ballentine, M.D. and Alan Hymes, M.D. *Science of Breath: A Practical Guide,* Honesdale, PA.   Himalayan International Institute of Yoga Science and Philosophy, 1979.

Ravizza, Richard. "The Nasal Wash- A Glance at the Research", *Yoga International Reprint Series- Inner Body Cleansing.* Honesdale, PA.: Himalayan International Institute of Yoga Science and Philosophy.

Shannahoff-Khalsa, David. "Breathing for the Brain," *American Health,* November, 1986. P. 16, 18.

Speads, Carola J. *Ways to Better Breathing.* Rochester, VT: Inner Traditions International Ltc., 1992.

van Lysebeth, Andre. *Pranayama- the Yoga of Breathing.* London. Unwin Paperbacks, 1983.

Videos

Hendricks, Gay Ph.D "Conscious Breathing," 1-800-688-0772

Coping with Stress : Yoga Style

> *There is a quiet, peaceful place, deep down inside each and every one of us, that can't be touched by the storms of life that swirl around us.*
> *Learn how to become friends with your quiet, peaceful, inner self.*
> . . . **Swami Rama, Founder of the Himalayan Institute of Yoga Science and Philosophy**

Yoga is recommended as an activity to help people cope with the stress in their life. As you will discover as you do yoga and read this unit, yoga incorporates into its approach.

1. <u>Exercise</u> : Which is always recommended for stress as it releases tension through physical activity
2. <u>Deep Breathing</u>: Which was discussed in unit 5
3. <u>Relaxation</u>: Which is done between the yoga asanas and at the end of a yoga session
4. <u>Imagery and Visualization</u>:   This is done by having the mind use scenes of nature or of the inner body to help bring about relaxation
5. <u>Music</u>: Which is used during relaxation to help with the freeing of the mind and body
6. <u>Meditation:</u> Which is taught based upon origins from yoga

Each of these techniques, along with some others, will be discussed in greater detail. First, a brief review of stress and its impact on the body.

STRESS

What Is It?

Stress was first identified by Hans Selye, a Hungarian who emigrated to the Unites States in 1931 and then moved to Toronto, Canada. In 1936, he published his first article about his research with rats. When the research rats had been deprived of their freedom and their diet altered, they exhibited ulcerated stomachs and a loss of fat content in their thymus gland (authors notes from Dr. Selye's lecture at Ball State University 1979). His research over the years has resulted in his authoring 38 books and 1760 scientific articles. Now, in one year, there are over 6,000 reports written concerning stress research.

Dr. Selye defines stress as "the non specific response of the body to any demand." This means that good and bad events can both cause stress. The word "eustress" refers to a good event, such as the excitement resulting from your team winning a close sporting event. "Distress" is the word used to describe the response from getting bad news about money or health. In both situations the body responds in a physical manner which is known as the "fight or flight response" (Table 6.1). These are normal responses of the body to protect it from harm coming from a potential enemy. This response should not be thought of in only a negative manner as it can function as a force that brings about a desire to create and accomplish a goal. We can let our incentive and growth be enhanced if we think of stress with this attitude. However, when the level of stress remains high for an extended period of time, the body can develop some disorders that can lead to health problems (Table 6.2).

Fight or Flight Response

- Breathing speeds up
- Perspiration increases
- Blood pressure raises
- Digestion stops
- Body can begin shaking
- Feel keyed up
- Heart rate increases
- Pupils dilate
- Muscles in arms and legs tense
- Blood goes to muscles
- Feel restless

Table 6.1

Some Stress-Related Disorders	
Accidents	Duodenal ulcer/colitis
Acne	Eczema
Alcoholism	Heartburn
Allergies	Hypertension
Asthma	Migraine headaches
Backache	Nervous tics
Chronic fatigue	Obesity
Coronary artery disease	Spastic colon
Depression	Sexual dysfunction in both men and women

Table 6.2

Dr. Selye thinks that there is a certain amount of energy available for our use throughout our life and that when this is used up we reach a stage of exhaustion and eventually die. Stress affects this level of resistance. He calls this concept the "General Adaptation Syndrome." The important thing to remember is that we can change the length of time that we stay in the "stage of resistance" by doing some stress coping activities. Thus, we preserve some of our life energy, PRANA   and do not reach the "exhaustion stage" where the stress related disorders begin appearing. In beginning to cope with stress it is important to be aware of your response to the stressor. **You** are in charge of how you perceive an event causing stress and **you** are responsible for your own emotional and physical response. Your perception of the event is under your control even if the event is not. Stress of one kind or another will always be with you so what can be of help is to identify what <u>causes</u> the stress for you by referring to the checklists in Appendix A and to discover effective ways to alleviate the stress by reading the next section.

WHAT CAN I DO TO HELP COPE WITH STRESS?

Physical Activity Combined With Relaxation

Dr. Selye has suggested that the person who exercises regularly is better able to resist the stressors in their life. Hatha yoga poses are ideal for this as they do not increase the stress on the body as some forms of exercise can do for some people. The yoga stretches have been referred to as "Mother Nature's Tranquilizer"- to stretch a muscle helps relax a muscle.

When doing yoga asanas, you are encouraged to work while you are doing the pose and then to" let go" when you have completed the exercise, allowing the body to go limp. You should feel the energy and thrill of the <u>doing</u> of the asana and then feel the <u>release</u>

of the tension as you allow yourself to relax between the asanas.

In yoga we do the complete relaxation pose, SAVASANA.   This Sanskrit word " SAVA" means "corpse" and you want the body to be as free of tension as it would be if it were a corpse. In India the belief in reincarnation is popular,therefore using the corpse for imagery is not upsetting to them. Our western minds are sometimes not as comfortable with this image so it is sometimes referred to as the "sponge" or as the "yoga relaxation pose."

There are several ways to reach this relaxed state. One technique, called "progressive relaxation," involves tensing a body part before giving it the cue to relax. Another approach is to talk to the body giving it cues without tensing the area. Both approaches work and it is usually a matter of personal preference, and/ or time, as to which method is used. Refer to Fig. 6.1 and follow these directions to achieve a stress free alignment for the body in SAVASANA.

Savasana:

Sitting with the knees bent, place your two fists between your knees. Look to make sure your feet are a little wider than your knees. Place your hands on top of your knees. Straighten your right leg and then your left leg so they form the letter "V." Slowly, as you lower your back to the mat, imagine that you are placing each vertebrae down one after the other. You are laying the spine on the floor as you would lay down a string of pearls. Next, bend your elbows, bring your fingertips up to touch the shoulders. Place the elbows next to your ribs and then slide them out about 3-4 inches. Straighten out your arms, bringing the lower arms down so that the palms are turned UP to the ceiling and you have your shoulderblades tucked slightly together. Now you are in your yoga relaxation position. Palms must be turned up. If the palms are turned down you will feel your shoulders leave the mat and thus not able to relax as completely.

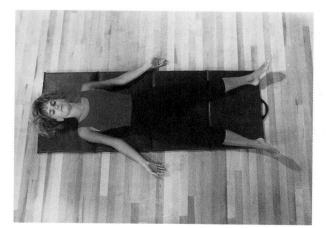

Figure 6.1   *Savasana*

The following are some adjustments you can make for greater comfort. If you have a lower back problem and it bothers your back to lie with your legs straight, bend your knees or place a pillow under your legs. If you are feeling tension in the neck or shoulders, turn your head slowly from side to side. When you bring it back to the center, visualize that the nose, chin and sternum are in a straight line.

Now that the body is correctly positioned, be aware of your breath and allow the body to totally relax. If you are feeling tension in any area of your body, take a moment to mentally suggest to that part of you to relax. Also suggest to your mind to relax by being aware of your breath or the relaxation music that may be playing.

At the end of your relaxation time follow these directions. Keeping the eyes closed, lift your arms up as you inhale, hook your thumbs together and stretch the arms over your head and lower them to the floor behind you. Turn onto your right side and move the body into a half moon with the arms and legs behind you, stretching the abdominal area. Then release that stretch and roll onto your back. Turn onto your left side and arch and stretch. Release to the back. Bend your knees with your feet flat on the mat, tilt the pelvis and then turn onto your right side. Place the left arm across your body, palm to the floor in front of the chest. Bend your right elbow slightly, and use your two hands to slowly push yourself up to a sitting position on the right thigh. Eyes are still closed. Sit with your legs crossed at the ankles and the back erect.

Now comes the "palming technique." Rub your hands together until they are nice and hot. Place the palms over your eyes.Open your eyes, slide the fingers apart to let in a little light and bring your hands down. This is a very gentle way to re-enter your environment.

Pranayama

> *It is certainly not the aim of breathing work,*
> *nor is it possible,*
> *to have one's breathing unaffected by life*
> *or to avoid life's problems.*
> *On the contrary, contact with your breathing will*
> *make you more open to life's experiences.*
> *. . . Carola H. Speads*

Unit 5 discussed the benefits and directions for yoga breathing. It is again mentioned here as a reminder that the breath has a calming effect on the body and can be practiced as a stress coping technique. While lying in the relaxation pose described above, practice the Yoga Complete Breath. Allow the entire chest and abdominal area to expand as you slowly inhale and then slowly control the exhale. Before meditation do the Alternate Nostril Breath. All of the PRANAYAMA techniques taught are beneficial.

Meditation

> *Without full awareness of breathing,*
> *there can be no development of*
> *meditative stability and understanding.*
>
> **—Thich Nhat Hanh**

What is meditation? It has been made to seem rather mysterious and sometimes controversial. It actually involves sitting quietly, allowing the body to become calm, taking deep breaths and allowing the mind to be still. Throughout history and in all parts of the world there are examples of "meditation." It is not something new that came out of the "hippy era." It can take the form of a simple prayer, of sitting alone on a beach watching the ocean or watching clouds on a mountaintop.

Meditation was practiced by the early Christian monks who were hermits living in the desert in the Fourth century; in the ancient Jewish tradition where the teachings of meditation were called Kabbalah; by the Moslems who also have a tradition of meditation; in the Hindu method which has been taught to many Westerners (Beatles included) by Maharishi Mahish Yogi and is known as TM - Trancendental Meditation; by Tibetan Buddhists and there is also the Zen tradition from Japan. All these approaches differ somewhat in their technique but the end result is similar in that the stilling of the body leads to the calming of the mind and the calming of the mind brings stress reduction benefits to the stilled body.

It is difficult to describe what can happen as everyone responds to meditation in their own way and develops a technique at their own pace. It is probably close to being asleep but at the same time being aware of your surroundings-you are in what is called the alpha state.

Following are some suggestions for meditating following the hatha yoga asanas, relaxation and PRANAYAMA:

1. Sit with hips elevated on a small pillow with the legs crossed, back erect, hands resting on the knees, eyes closed and   head level
2. Allow the mind to be quiet- forget the past, present, and the future
3. Regulate your breath for 5 minutes by exhaling on a count of 3-4 and inhaling on a count of 3-4
4. Allow the mind to wander for awhile. Do not FORCE it to be still
5. Focus on your breath or on a word that you like such as LOVE, PEACE, JOY or the Sanskrit word OHM
6. You can also focus between your eyebrows at the "mind's eye" or at the heart's center
7. Stay calm and don't force yourself. ENJOY
8. 20 minutes is fine but longer is all right too

Considerable research has been done using meditation techniques as a therapy for a variety of illness. For more information refer to the discussion in Unit 9, Therapeutic Use of Yoga.

Biofeedback

> *Meditation means first self analysis,*
> *then self cultivation, then self development,*
> *then self unfoldment, and then self enlightenment.*
> *Meditation is self-knowledge.*
> ... Swami Rama
> . . . Swami by Doug Boyd

The definition of the word, BIOFEEDBACK, simply means that the signals from your own body are listened to by YOU. In 1970, scientists at the Menninger Foundation Research Department in Topeka, Kansas, collaborated with Swami Rama, a yoga teacher from India. He was asked to serve a year as a consultant to their Voluntary Controls Project. Here he demonstrated precise control over his autonomic nervous system and brain. The findings of this research increased the understanding of humans' ability to develop this control for themselves. This contributed to the development of electronic machines that inform a person when they are developing the technique of tuning in to themselves. These machines and hand held thermometers are used now by physical therapists, counsellors and psychologists, dentists and

nurses to aid in the treatment of their patients. The following are conditions where biofeedback is being used: to alleviate migraine and tension headaches, epilepsy, cardiac arrhythmias, high and low blood pressure, paralysis and other movement disorders, and digestive tract problems.

The basic step in using biofeedback is doing the relaxation that allows the "Fight or Flight" responses to abate. It is thought that biofeedback works because the patient knows they are relaxed by the information received from a machine that reads change in skin temperature or muscle tension. The signal received is like a reward for having achieved the relaxed state and they then received this "feedback." When doing yoga with awareness and breath, you are training yourself to develop this feedback system internally. If you should need biofeedback training to help you through a health situation, refer to the resources section for addresses of those to contact.

It is interesting to note that at the Himalayan Institute in Honesdale, PA., established by Swami Rama in the l970's, they now offer a biofeedback profile to let people know how well they are doing their yoga breath and relaxation. We have come full circle as the biofeedback machines are now giving "feedback" to yoga practioners. Instructions to improve your breathing and relaxation are then available if desired.

Music

> *Healing with music, voice, and sound*
> *is among the oldest and*
> *most holistic of medical approaches.*
> Richard Leviton ... *Yoga Journal*, Jan/Feb 1994

One of the prominent researchers in the use of music to lower stress is Steve Halpern, Ph.D. As a musician and a composer he noticed changes in himself when he played the trumpet and guitar in his jazz fusion band, and when, after meditating he played the piano freestyle. When he played freestyle the music was flowing, gentle and with no beat. Since his first interest in l969 he has become one of the leaders in the growth of "New Age Music." "My work has shown me that music can be not only a source of pleasure and entertainment but also a tool for reducing stress and improving our well being. In fact we can create music specifically aimed at making our lives balanced and peaceful" (*The l989 Guide to New Age Living,*p. 62-64." Musical Meditation" by Steve Halpern).

He returned to graduate school at Sonoma State University and conducted research using his compositions and classical music, measuring the subjects' responses to each by using Kirlian photography (high frequency, high voltage electrophotography developed by the Russians that produced a picture of the energy field that surrounds the physical body the "aura"); electroencephalogram (measuring brain waves); and Galvanic skin response (electrical resistance on the surface of the the skin). No matter what technique was used, the music of Steve Halpern produced a "statistically significant" effect on a wide variety of subjects. For example, the brain waves would be in the beta range (13-39 cycles per second) for classical music and in the alpha range (8-12 cycles per second) for the new age music.

As reported in the book *Healthy Pleasures*, by Robert Ornstein Ph.D., and David Sobel, M.D., research conducted in California, Japan and West Germany has led to discoveries that indicate that:

- Music stimulates the release of endorphins, like chemicals that the brain produces
- The beat of the music will cause the heart to speed up or slow down
- The electrical rhythms of the brain are altered
- Slower, quiet music, with no singing, lowers blood pressure and slows respiration
- Soothing music played before, during and after surgery in operating rooms reduces the level of stress hormones in the blood
- Music played in coronary care units reduces heart rates, loweres blood pressure, lessens depression and increases tolerance for pain
- During childbirth among women trained in the Lamaze technique music reduced pain and shortened labor by two hours
- Music therapy may be helpful with premature infants, autistic children, cancer, stroke, arthritic, diabetic and coma patients
- In healthy people it is thought that the function of the immune system is enhanced by music

For those who have a growing interest in Sound/Music Therapy there are two national organization for Music Therapy. The addresses are listed in the resources at the end of this unit. These organizations compile the research findings and report to their membership. More ways of helping people heal themselves through music are continuing to emerge. For example, a woman who had not recovered the use of her leg following hip replacement surgery found the leg responding with movement to Irish Jig music. A person with Parkinson's disease (neurological disor-

der) who could not initiate any movement and whose posture would remain fixed in an awkward position for days was able to "put her hands on a piano keyboard and 'she can play beautifully and for hours-and when she plays her Parkinsonism disappears and all is ease and fluency and freedom and normality,' claims her doctor, Oliver Sacks, M.D." (Leviton, *Yoga Journal,* Jan./Feb 1994, p. 61).

It is now a practice for infants to be welcomed at birth to soothing sounds and also to listen to audiotapes of the internal sounds of the mother that they were hearing as a fetus. What is now available to patients at St. Patrick's Hospital, Missoula, Montana, is "Music for Dying." A harpist, Therese Schroeder-Sheker, is training twenty students to bring their live harp music and human voice to the bedside of those who are taking their last breaths. Schroeder-Sheker says " this is probably the only hospital in the world with 27 harps and resident singing harpists-in-training" (Leviton,*Yoga Journal* , Jan/Feb. 1994. p. 125). These musicians are helping people face the transition between life and death with dignity and acceptance in a peaceful environment. It is now possible for the human to enter the world and depart with the calming effect of music creating an environment of peace.

There are many individuals who have contributed to this growing field of music therapy by composing music and combining sounds from nature with musical instruments to produce this "New Age " music, or "Space Music" as it is sometimes called. Don Campbell collaborated with the Simontons to make the first Music Therapy tape used in cancer treatment-"Symphony for the Inner Self." He is the founder/director of the Institute for Music, Health and Education in Boulder, Colorado . Campbell's approach is to awaken the inner musician in his clients. I have been at workshops conducted by Jean Houston, Ph.D., with the music provided by Don Campbell and it is always an experience that goes deep and one you will never forget.

It is most often in a yoga class or a massage session that people are first exposed to this wonderful music that greatly facilitates a state of relaxation. For an example of how society has accepted the concept of sound therapy, read on. We now have available for purchase the "Heart and Sound Soother" from one of the respected electronic wizardy stores. By pressing a button you can chose 1. heartbeat to sooth infants, 2. gentle patter of rain, 3. a gurgling brook, 4. neutral white noise to screen out background noise, 5. ocean waves, or 6. sounds of a summer night. This machine has been designed to operate on batteries and electricity. You are invited to consult the resource list for names and addresses for obtaining music for relaxation and/or meditation. There are publications that discuss this type of music and the artists that perform it.

Imagery and Visualization

> *When one's thoughts are neither*
> *frivolous nor flippant,*
> *when one's thoughts are neigher*
> *stiff-necked nor stupid,*
> *but rather, are harmonious-*
> *they habitually render physical calm*
> *and deep insight.*
> **Hildegarde of Bingen, Benedictine Abbess (1098-1179)**

When you are relaxing in the yoga pose of SAVASANA (corpse) it is a perfect time to do visualization. You can create in your mind's eye a beautiful setting in nature such as a mountain top, under your favorite tree or by the ocean, allowing your mind to recreate the sounds, sights, feel of the breeze, warmth of the sun, or the smell of the ocean, flowers or pine tree. This will have a calming effect on you and will allow your mind to center in on this pleasant task. You will almost feel that you are really there in this special place you have created. With your mind involved in creating this inner environment it can not think of your other concerns or problems.

Dr. William Fezler, a psychotherapist, has used imagery with over 3,000 patients to help them with conditions that ranged from alcoholism to anxiety attacks. His book, *Creative Imagery; How to Visualize in All Five Senses,* is easy to follow and contains little scenarios that he has composed that you can read to yourself or use for ideas to create your own imagery. He states, that "Images-what you imagine-possess not only the power to heal, but to take you to higher realms of knowledge and experience than you've ever visited" (Introduction p. ix).

This connection between the brain and the body is becoming more widely recognized. It is discussed in popular magazines as well as researched in respected centers of learning such as Harvard, Yale, and Duke Universities. The applications of this emerging field of study range from simply practicing positive thinking to the intense mental practice used by Olympic athletes to perfect their skills. It is recommended that you use this imagery or mental practice in your daily life. Allow some time in your day to

develop this technique. Perhaps it may involve learning a new skill such as typing or the use of computers, or a sports skill such as your tennis or golf swing. This technique is also part of the approach taken in the many self-healing programs and books that have appeared in recent years. Dr. Carl Simonton and his wife Stephanie Matthews Simonton, Bernard Siegal M.D., Jon Kabatt-Zin M.D., and Norman Cousins have all made use of this approach and similar ones to help people in situations of chronic pain and terminal illness. They all have written books that are listed in the resources at the end of this unit or unit 9.

To further the study of the mind/body in a scientific manner, the Institute for the Advancement of Health was established in 1983. The institute publishes a scholarly journal, *Advances,* and funds research projects dealing with brain and immune system interactions; stress and health; and behavioral and psychological treatments for medical disorders. This institute is now known as the FEZLER Institute and were the sponsors of the highly popular and acclaimed *"Healing and the Mind "* PBS television series that is discussed in Unit 9.

An astronaut from the Apollo 14 flight to the moon, Edgar Mitchell, founded a non-profit organization, Institue of Noetic Sciences, in 1973. This Institute also funds research projects in the emerging field of psychoneuroimmunology (see resources). In 1991, they published *The Noetic Sciences Collection: 1980-1990 Ten Years of Consciousness Research.* This publication has reprints of the previously printed articles which covered topics from imagery in sports, "Healing, Remission and Miracle Cures," and " On Meditation and the Western Mind, " to "Energy Medicine in China." The future will undoubtedly bring further findings and a greater understanding of the complicated and important mind/body connection.

Chakras

One of the branches of yoga that is known as KUNDALINI, is concerned with the flow of the energy through the body. There are seven chakras (see Fig. 6.2) beginning at the base of the spine, #1, and ending at the crown of the head, #7. It is thought that these energy centers correspond with areas of the body and also with psychological traits. It is also believed that these centers respond to a <u>sound</u> vibration in a therapeutic manner. In Western medicine "ultra sound" (sound vibration) is now used in a variety of ways to help with health conditions.

Also <u>color</u> is used with the chakras when meditating. These colors follow the spectrum of the

Figure 6.2   *Chakra System*

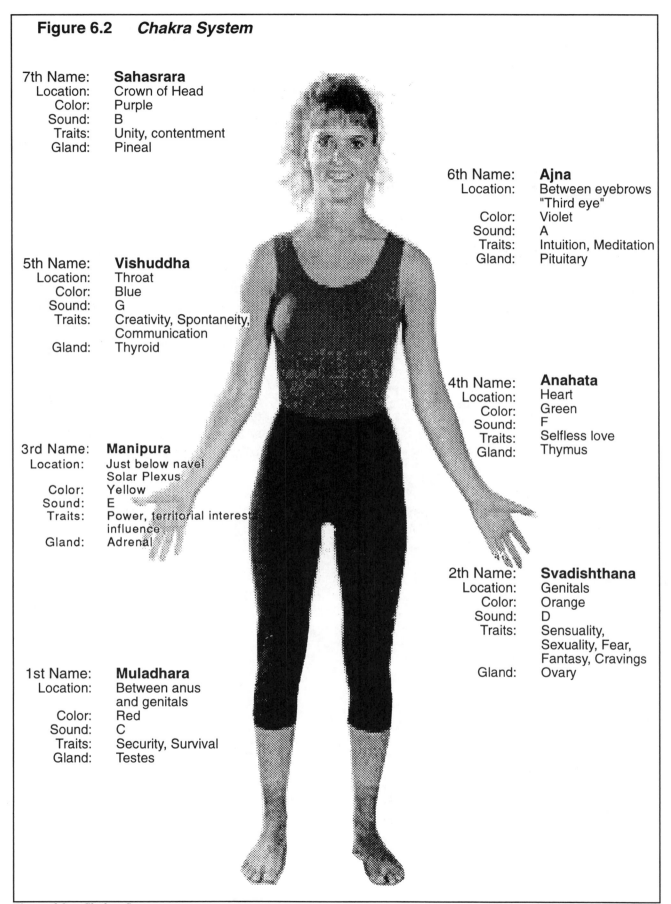

7th Name: **Sahasrara**
Location: Crown of Head
Color: Purple
Sound: B
Traits: Unity, contentment
Gland: Pineal

6th Name: **Ajna**
Location: Between eyebrows
"Third eye"
Color: Violet
Sound: A
Traits: Intuition, Meditation
Gland: Pituitary

5th Name: **Vishuddha**
Location: Throat
Color: Blue
Sound: G
Traits: Creativity, Spontaneity,
Communication
Gland: Thyroid

4th Name: **Anahata**
Location: Heart
Color: Green
Sound: F
Traits: Selfless love
Gland: Thymus

3rd Name: **Manipura**
Location: Just below navel
Solar Plexus
Color: Yellow
Sound: E
Traits: Power, territorial interest
influence
Gland: Adrenal

2th Name: **Svadishthana**
Location: Genitals
Color: Orange
Sound: D
Traits: Sensuality,
Sexuality, Fear,
Fantasy, Cravings
Gland: Ovary

1st Name: **Muladhara**
Location: Between anus
and genitals
Color: Red
Sound: C
Traits: Security, Survival
Gland: Testes

Figure 6.2   *Chakra System*

rainbow as you move up the spine. Working with KUDALINI energy is said to affect your consciousness and your attitudes, motives, mental state and relationships.

The Fig. 6.2 provides more basic information about this theory. Whole books are written on this aspect of yoga. For more information refer to the resource section. It is recommended that this aspect of yoga is best practiced under the guidance of a teacher.

Flotation Tanks

> *The water had a pleasant viscosity.*
> *I felt like a chunk of Dole pineapple*
> *in a dish of slowly congealing Jell-O*
> ... Marc Barasch,
> Editorial *New Age Journal*. May '84.

This form of relaxation has its origins in the early 1970s, when John Lilly M.D., a neuroscientist who had become famous working with the communications skills of dolphins, set up a tank of water at the National Institute of Mental Health. The tank is designed so there is no sound or light and you float in about 10 inches of 93.5°water that has 500-800 pounds of dissolved epsom salt. In this state of "sensory deprivation " the physical body can become totally relaxed once you learn to trust the buoyancy of the water. Then your mind can begin to relax and do interesting things. Some people have described their experience as "events" that flash on a "television screen" such as ideas, emotions, childhood memories and images that come and go. The sound of your own breathing and stomach gurgles is amazingly loud at the beginning, but as you calm down those sounds also become quieter. The time, usually an hour, goes by quickly. When the sound of New Age music coming out the speakers in the tank signals the end of your session, you are amazed and don't want to leave.

So what are the benefits? You will have the feeling of being relaxed, recharged and more alert to all the sensory input in the world such as sound, sense of touch and sight. Scientists such as Peter Suedfield of University of British Columbia and Thomas Fine of Medical College of Ohio, have found that there is an enhancement of learning, IQ scores, visual concentration, recall and perceptual motor tasks. Physically it has been found that endorphins are released and there is also a lowering of blood pressure and the stress -related biochemicals in the blood of those with hypertension (high blood pressure).

The tanks are now being used by athletes (Philadelphia Phillies won the World Series immediately after starting to use the tanks and the Philadelphia Eagles won the Super Bowl); by students to help enhance their learning of chemistry, languages etc; by physicians who recommend it to lower blood pressure, speed healing of broken bones, enhance recovery from heart surgery; by psychiatrists to help patients relieve phobias, depression, anxiety and stress; and by creative artists, writers and musicians who use it to tap into their creativity.

Flotation tanks are one invention of our technological society that allows us to enter a site of tranquility and peace and to allow a renewal of our body and spirit if desired (see Fig. 6.3).

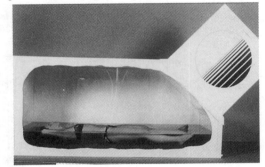

Figure 6.3   *Flotation Tank*

Following are some tips for enjoying and benefitting from your "float".

BEFORE:

Eat lightly before floating

Do not shave body hair that day to prevent any nicks which the salt could irritate

Shower before entering the tank

Put vaseline on any skin abrasions to keep salt out

Put ear plugs in your ears

You may want to wear a swim or shower cap

Place your towel where you can easily find it with your eyes closed

IN TANK:

Locate and practice opening the door before lying back in the water

Take deep breaths while in the tank

Find the sides so you know the space of your environment in the tank

Experiment with how you place your hands out to the side, behind neck, folded on chest or stomach. Move them slowly so you don't drip the salt water on your face

Allow yourself to relax and don't hold your head up

ENJOY!!!!

AFTER:

Take several deep breaths to start to energize your body

Hold head tilted back when you first sit up to keep the salty hair dripping down your back and not your face

Don't open your eyes until you have a towel to wipe around hair and face

Shower and shampoo thoroughly

Have a tablet and a pen to take notes about your experience

Do not plan a day full of activities following your float

Laughter

We all enjoy a good laugh and the cleansing and exhausted feeling we have following a bout of the giggles. And now researchers have discovered just how good laughter really is. In the following Table 6.3 there is a list of the body's responses to laughter. We began to take note of these benefits when Norman Cousins wrote a book, *Anatomy of an Illness*, (1979) that was a chronicle of his bout with a disease of the connective tissue. He watched old "slapstick movies" and discovered that "ten minutes of genuine belly laughter provided at least two hours of pain free sleep without medication."

BODY'S RESPONSE TO LAUGHTER

HEART: Doubles the rate for 3-5 minutes in only 20 seconds. Pumps greater amount of blood. Blood pressure rises temporarily.

LUNGS: Ventilation is enhanced as you expel more of the residual air that stays in lungs between a normal breath. This allows more oxygen rich air to be inhaled and you get rid of a greater amount of carbon dioxide

ENDOCRINE GLANDS: ADRENALINE is released and triggers the pituitary gland to release ACTH (adrenocorticotropic hormone) which stimulates the kidneys to secrete CORTISOL. The bodys natural painkiller, ENDORPHIN is then released. The body produces more immune cells

MUSCULAR and SKELETAL SYSTEM: Muscles of the scalp, face, neck, shoulders, chest and abdomen get a workout. Following laughter there is a reduction of muscle tension. Arms and legs also can get involved.

METABOLISM: Accelerates and it is estimated that you burn 78 times as many calories as you do when you are at rest. This is known as "Inner Jogging."

I imagine you are wondering how laughter fits into a yoga class. The following Crocodile Routine (Table 6.4) was developed by a yoga teacher from India, Swami Dev Murti, and was taught to the English in the 1960's. This routine incorporates laughter at steps 9a and 9b. The whole routine is very beneficial, especially for the back, which will be discussed in Unit 9. The International Yoga Centre in Kent, which was established by Swami Dev Murti, is a delightful place to stay and to enjoy this style of yoga. Refer to the resource section for the address of this center.

CROCODILE ROUTINE

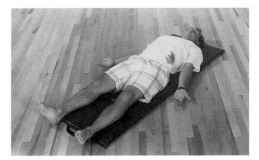

Figure 6.4A   *Basic Body Position*

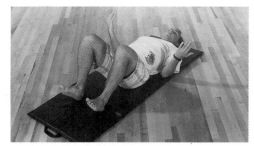

Figure 6.4B   *Fish Relaxation*

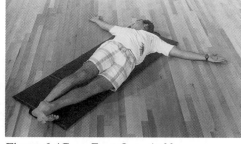

Figure 6.4C   *Foot Over Ankle*

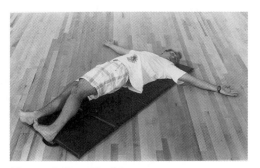

Figure 6.4D   *Heel Between Big Toe and Second Toe*

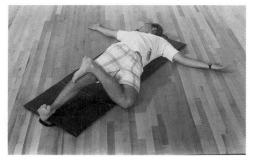

Figure 6.4E   *Ankle on Top of Knee of Other Leg*

BASIC BODY POSITION : (Fig. 6.4A) Lie on the back with legs straight and feet together. Arms stretched out sideways level with the shoulders and palms up. Inhale- Push breath down to abdominal cavity. Twist turning the head to the right and the body to the left. Slowly roll from side to side as long as breath can be held. Exhale and follow with the -

FISH RELAXATION:(Fig. 6.4B) Arms down by sides, bend knees and elbows slightly as you inhale and let them drop and flop as you exhale. Do 3 times.

1. **Right** foot crosses over the **left** ankle. Keep shoulders on floor on all of the twists.
   FISH RELAXATION

2. **Left** foot over the **right** ankle. Twist (Fig. 6.4C)
   FISH RELAXATION

3. **Right** heel between big toe and next toe of **left** foot. Twist (Fig. 6.4D)
   FISH RELAXATION

4. **Left** heel between big toe and next toe of **right** foot. Twist
   FISH RELAXATION

5. Bend **right** knee and place the outside of the **right** ankle on top (Fig. 6.4E) of the **left** knee and twist keeping shoulders on the floor.
   FISH RELAXATION

6. Bend **left** knee and place the outside of the **left** ankle on top of the **right** knee and twist keeping shoulders on the floor.
   FISH RELAXATION

7. a. Bend knees, place feet flat and as close to buttocks as possible. Separate feet and knees so that when twisting the **right** knee touches the floor next to the **left** heel and vice versa (Fig. 6.4F).
FISH RELAXATION

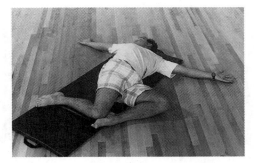

Figure 6.4F   *Knees Bent and Legs Apart*

b. Feet and knees together when twisting this time. The top foot rests on the side of the bottom foot (Fig. 6.4G)

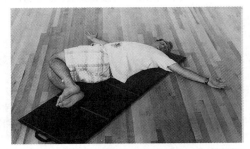

Figure 6.4G   *Knees Bent and Legs Together*

8. a. Knees to chest and clasp hands behind knees and then roll from side to side with the head going opposite of the knees (Fig. 6.4H).
FISH RELAXATION

b. Knees to chest and roll back onto shoulders and up to a sitting position (Fig. 6.4I).
FISH RELAXATION

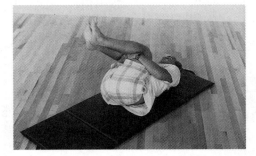

Figure 6.4H   *Knees to Chest and Rolling*

9. a. Basic position but you add a cycling movement with the arms and legs as you laugh loudly on each vowel: HA, HE, HI, HO, HU. Take a new breath for each vowel and laugh until all the air has been expired (Fig. 6.4I).
FISH RELAXATION

b. With the body lying in basic position, laugh with the mouth closed so the air comes out through the nose only.
FISH RELAXATION

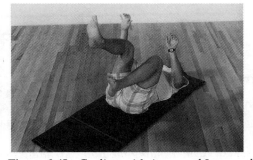

Figure 6.4I   *Cycling with Arms and Legs and Laughing*

10. In basic position link the fingers and turn hands so palms are toward the feet. **Inhale** and slowly with tension on the arm move the hands toward the chest skimming the body surfaceuntil you need to **exhale**. Repeat 2 more times (Fig. 6.4J).
FISH RELAXATION

11. Arms over head with hands linked, roll several times to right and left.
FISH RELAXATION

12. Sitting up with legs crossed do shoulder rolls:

  a. Both forward and both back
  b. Right forward and left back
  c. Left forward and right back
  d. Both up and both down
  e. One up and one down.
  FISH RELAXATION

13. Deep Relaxation. SAVASANA

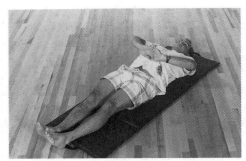

Figure 6.4J   *Fingers Linked - Palms Toward Feet*

Following are some suggestions on how to add humor and laughter to your daily life.

- Surround yourself with people who are fun and who will make you laugh
- Look for humor around you
- Laugh at yourself
- Have cartoons and funny quotes handy so you can see them and laugh
- Do the laughter step 9a and 9b (page 91) when you need a good laugh
- Watch a funny movie when you are not feeling well

SUMMARY

Stress is a part of our lives and the best way to deal with it is to recognize its presence and do one or more of the activities suggested in this unit to help alleviate it. Also try some of the following tips to help you deal with stress.

Slow down and admire nature and the change of season.
Do one thing at a time
Give yourself time to finish a task
Sometimes slow down your speaking, eating and walking
Take your watch off on the weekends
Take time each day for some form of relaxing:float tank, listening to music, meditating
Sing whenever you feel like it
DON'T feel guilty about relaxing- you deserve it
Do something for someone else who is "stressed out" and you both will benefit
Listen to your body and know when you are pushing too hard
Try to get enough sleep and follow good eating habits
Remember how YOU react to stress is under your control!

RESOURCES

Physical Activity and Relaxation

Benson, Herbert and Miriam Z Klipper. *The Relaxation Response.* New York, NY: Avon Books, 1979.
_____."Beyond Relaxation- The Renewable Mind," *American Health-Fitness of Body and Mind.* Sept 1987, p 76-83.
Borysenko, Joan. *Minding the Body, Mending the Mind.* New York, NY.: Bantam, 1987.
_____ "Love is the Healer," *Yoga Journal,* May/June 1990. p. 45-49,94, 98.
_____. *Guilt is the Teacher, Love is the Lesson.* New York, NY.: Warner, 1990.
Crooks, Cheryl. "Can a Mineral Mitigate Stress?" *American Health-Fitness of Body and Mind.* June, 1985, p. 112.
Goleman, Daniel, and Tara Bennett Goleman. *American Health's Relaxed Body Book.* New York: Doubleday. 1986.
_____ "Moving Toward Mindfullness," *American Health-Fitness of Body and Mind,* March 1987, p. 80-88.
Lasater, Judith Hanson. " 10 Ways to Relax Deeply," *Yoga Journal.* Jan/Feb. 1992. p. 75-81.
_____"Relax and Renew," *Yoga Journal.* October, 1995. p. 74-83.
Ornstein, Robert Ph.D, and David Sobel M.D. *Healthy Pleasures.* Reading, MA: Addison-Wesley Publishing Co.Inc. 1989.
Pelletier, Kenneth R. *Mind as Healer, Mind as Slayer: A Holistic Approach to Preventing Stress Disorders.* New York: Dell, 1977.
Quyle, P.A. "Yoga on The Run," *Working Mother.* Vol 15, June, 1992. p. 22.

Selye, Hans. *Stress Without Distress.* New York. Signet, 1974.
Siegel, Bernie S. M.D. *Love, Medicine and Miracles.*   New York, NY: Harper and Row, Publishers. 1990
_____ *Peace, Love and Healing.* New York, NY: Harper and Row, Publishers. 1989.

Pranayama

Iyengar, B.K.S. *Light on Pranayama.* New York, Crossroad Publishing Co., 1981.
Swami Rama, Rudolph Ballentine, M.D., and Alan Hymes, M.D. *Science of the Breath.* Honesdale, PA: Himalayan
     Publishers. 1995.

Meditation

Ballentine, Rudolph, M.D. *The Theory and Practice of Meditation.* Honesdale, PAHimalayan Publishers. 1986.
Christensen, Alice. *The American Yoga Association Beginner's Manual.* New York: Simon & Shuster, Inc.
     A Fireside Book, 1987.
Kornfield, Jack , Ph.D. "On Meditation and the Western Mind,".*Noetic Sciences Collection: 1980-1990
Ten Years of Consciousness Research.* Sausalito CA: The Institute of Noetic Sciences, 1991, p.117-123.
Schoefield, G. "Meditations What You Need; The Virtues of Yoga for Patients and Nurses,"
     Nursing Standard (English) May, 1994, p. 18-24.

Biofeedback

The Biofeedback Society of America, 4301 Owens Street, Wheat Ridge, CO 80033. (303)422-8436. Maintains a
     network of State societies.
The Biofeedback Certification Institute of America, 4301, Owens Street, Wheat Ridge,CO 80033 (303)420-2902.
     Provides national certification.
For inexpensive temperature feedback devices:
     Echo, Inc. P.O.Box 87, Springfield, OH 45501, (513) 322-4972.
     Bio-temp Products, Inc., 1950 W. 86th St., Indianapolis, IN 46260, (317) 872-9888.
HIMALAYAN INSTITUTE, RR1, Honesdale, PA 18431. 1-800-444-5772.

Music
Articles:
Halpern, Steve Ph.D. "Musical Meditation,"*The 1989 Guide to New Age Living*,p. 62-64.
Leviton, Richard. "Healing Vibrations," *Yoga Journal,* Jan/Feb. 1994 p. 59-64.
     "Body and Soul Music," *American Health-Fitness ofBody and Mind,* June, 1985,p.66-67.
"Soul Music," *New Age Journal,* April 1987, p. 58-63.

Catalogs:
Institute for Music, Health and Education. Director; Don G. Campbell, P.O Box 1244, Boulder, CO 80306.
Heartbeats, from Backroads Distributors, 417 Tamal Plaza, Corte Madera, CA 94925 1-800-825-4848.
Heartsong Review, PO Box 1084, Cottage Grove OR 97424. This is a published twice a year as a resource guide for
     new age music as well as a catalog. Two-year subscription- $10.00. One-year is $6.00.

Audio Tapes:
Campbell, Don. "Angels," "Crystal Rainbows," "Crystal Meditations," "Cosmic Classics."
Enya. "Watermark," "Enya," "Shephards Moon."
Halpern, Steve. "Dawn," "Spectrum Suite," "Crystal Suite," "Gaia's Groove." and Georgia Kelly, "Ancient Echos."
Rowland, Mike. "The Fairy Ring," "Solace," "Titania," and "Silver Wings."
Solitude Series. Nature Soundtracks- birds, swamps, lakes, oceans.
Environments Series. Oceans, meadows, forests, thunderstorm, sailboat and ocean.
Horn, Paul. "Inside the Pyramids," "Inside the Taj Mahal," "Peace Album"- Christmas.
Lanz, David. "Christofori's Dream."
Vollenweider, Andreas. "Caverna Magica," "Behind the Garden...," "Dancing With the Lion," "Down to the Moon."

Organizations:

American Association for Music Therapy, P.O. Box 80012, Valley Forge, PA 19484   (315) 265-4006.

National Association for Music Therapy, 8455 Colesville Rd., Ste. 930, Silver Springs, MD 20910, (301) 589-3300.

Imagery
Publications:

Advances, Journal of Mind-Body Health, The Fetzer Institute, 9292 West KL Ave., Kalamazoo, MI 49009
        (616)375-2000.

Fezler, William. *Creative Imagery: How to Visualize in All Five Senses.* New York, NY; Fireside Book. Simon &
        Shuster Inc. 1989.

Gawain, Shakti. *Creative Visualization.*   New York: Bantam Books,1978.

Institute of Noetic Sciences; P.O. Box 909, Sausalito, CA 94966-0909 (415) 331-5650.

Kabat-Zin, Jon MD *Wherever You Go, There You are: Mindfulness Meditation in Everyday Life.*
        New York. Hyperion, 1994.

Marrone, Robert. *Body of Knowledge: An Introduction to Body/Mind Psychology,*
        Albany N.Y. State University of New York Press. 1990.

Miller, D. Patrick. "Where Scientists and Mystics Meet," *Yoga Journal,* September/October, 1989. p.63-66.

Brain Mind Bulletin. Editor/publisher Marilyn Ferguson, Interface Press, Box 2211, 4717 N. Figueroa St.,
        Los Angeles CA 90042.

Video Tapes:

Halpern, Steven. "Summer Wind" 35 minutes.

Halpern, Steven, and other musicians. "Natural Light: Windance". 30 minutes

Floating

Hutchison, Michael. "Exploring the Inner Sea," *New Age Journal.* May, 1984, p. 37-43.

_____. *The Book of Floating.* New York, NY: William Morrow and Company, 1984.

Chakras
Audio Tape:

Grof, Christina, *"Kundalina."*

Video Tape:

MacLaine, Shirley. "Inner Workout."

Books:

"Seven Levels of Consciousness." *Psychology Today.* December 1975.

Iyengar, B.K.S. *Light on Yoga,* New York: Schocken Books, 1965.

Smith, Bob and Linda Boudreau -Smith *Yoga for a New Age.* Englewood Cliffs, New Jersey: Prentice-Hall, Inc.

Laughter

Cousins,Norman. *Anatomy of an Illness.* New York. W.W. Norton & Co., 1979.

Peter, Lawrence J.   *The Laughter Prescription.* New York, NY: Ballantine, 1982.

International Yoga Centre, "Highfield," Lenham, Nr. Maidstone, Kent ME172EX England. Telephone: Lenham
        431 (858431).

Yoga: Nutrition & Weight Management

> *Your food shall be your medicine*
> *Your medicine shall be your food*
> . . . Hippocrates 424 B.C.

During the twenty-plus years that I have been a yoga teacher, I have observed that the students' interest in nutrition grows as *they* grew in their yoga practice. As they became more aware of their body through doing the yoga asanas, they gained respect for their body and its various complex functions. One of these functions being the connection between the food intake, weight management and the effect of appropriate nutrients, chemicals, and additives on their body. Over the years the students and I have discussed some of the current trends, fad diets and old established nutrition choices. Since I am not a trained nutritionist, I don't pretend to have all the answers but discuss the basics and make suggestion of where to go for more information. I have observed a heightened awareness of the importance of good nutrition habits in the students' lives. Following is a discussion of nutrition related topics that is of interest to the hatha yoga students.

NATIONAL DIETARY GUIDELINES

In 1980 the "Dietary Guidelines for Americans" were established by the United States Department of Agriculture and the United States Department of Health, Education and Welfare, now called the Department of Health and Human Services. These were reviewed and in 1985 the following guidelines were agreed upon:

- Eat a variety of foods
- Maintain desirable weight
- Avoid too much fat, saturated fat and cholesterol
- Eat foods adequate in starch and fiber
- Avoid too much sugar
- Avoid too much sodium
- If you drink alcohol, do so in moderation

The following table can be a helpful reference as it suggests an average daily caloric intake, the maximum advisable calories from fat, grams of fat, and milligrams of sodium for children, adult males and females.

	Age	Average Daily Calorie Intake	Maximum Calories From Fat	Fat Grams	Milligrams of Sodium
Children	7-10	2400	500		
Females	11-18	2200	450	44	1100 to 3300
	19-50	2100	400		for adults
	51- up	1800	350		(pregnant women
					need more-see MD)
Males	11-18	2700	650	67	
	19-50	2800	600		
	51-up	2400	500		

Table 7.1

FOOD PYRAMID + WATER

One of the basic nutrition recommendations is to eat a variety of foods so that you are meeting all of your nutritional needs. The following table is based on the recommended daily servings from the US Government's Food Pyramid.

RECOMMENDED DAILY NUTRITION NEEDS FOR ADULTS		
Grains	6-11	servings daily
Vegetables & Beans	4-6	servings daily
Fruits	2-4	servings daily
Dairy, Yogurt	2-3	servings daily
Fish, Poultry, Meat Nuts, Legumes	1-2	servings daily

Protein, which we obtain from fish, poultry, meat & legumes, is needed to build and repair the body. Carbohydrates, found in the beans, grains, nuts, and some vegetables provide us with our major source of energy. Fiber, vitamins and minerals are the other necessary ingredients for a healthy diet.

Water is an often neglected ingredient when discussing nutrition. When exercising, the circulation to the muscles increases and sweating will also occur. Thus the need for water is increased, as it will help rid the body of waste. Water also helps relieve constipation. Eight glasses a day are recommended and even more is all right. Bottled water is sometimes necessary when the local water source is known to be impure but watch the sodium content. It should be less than 60 mg per liter.

CENTER FOR SCIENCE IN THE PUBLIC INTEREST

This organization, CSPI, was developed as a consumer group to monitor the food industry and also to make recommendations to protect the health of the consumer. They publish a newsletter "Nutrition Action Health Letter," have published books and have also developed posters that have information about salt, sugar, fat and chemical content in food. There is also a version of the Food Pyramid that categorizes the foods as those to eat ANYTIME, SOMETIMES, and SELDOM. This division by categories is based on what are the most nutritious and what are the nutritional shortcomings. Refer to Table 7.3 for the ANYTIME recommendations which are low in fat and saturated fat, sodium, and sugar and have no other serious nutrition flaws such as dangerous chemical additives.

Jane Brody, a writer for the New York Times, when asked about nutritional references is quoted as having said "My personal favorite is *Nutrition Action."* Her food and fitness column is read by thousands. Michael Jacobson, the director of CSPI since its conception in the early 1970s, has been a guest on many talk shows and on national news sharing nutrition information with the consumer. One of this group's most valuable contributions has been the demand for and the development of food labeling. Learn to read labels so you know what you are ingesting in the way of hidden fat, sugar, salt and chemicals. When possible, make choices that supply your body with the most nutritional benefits offered.

SUPPLEMENTS TO FOOD INTAKE

Commercial Diet Centers and Eating Plans

These centers which develop an eating programs for a client may serve a purpose for those who are extremely obese. It is recommended that they be utilized with a physicians supervision. These can be very expensive programs as many of them require you to purchase ready made meals from them. One of the goals is to change the eating habits to what is recommended in the "Dietary Guidelines for Americans." For those who are slightly over weight or are of a normal weight they are not recommended.

Vitamins and Mineral Supplements

Professional nutritionists state that if you are eating the recommended daily servings from the Food Pyramid, it is not necessary to take vitamin and minerals in a tablet or pill form. But many people, depending on their work schedule, budget, where they are living (residence hall, sharing an apartment, or living with parents) do not always meet those daily recommendations. So examine your lifestyle and your present eating habits to see what **YOU** are doing. You don't want to waste your money on "expensive urine," as nutritionists suggest that is what happens with the water soluble vitamins (C and B complex). If more of the fat soluble vitamins (A,D, E and K) are taken into the body than you use, they will be stored and can cause health problems. Check with a physician and nutritionist about this concern. Vitamins and minerals such as calcium and iron, are important to the body

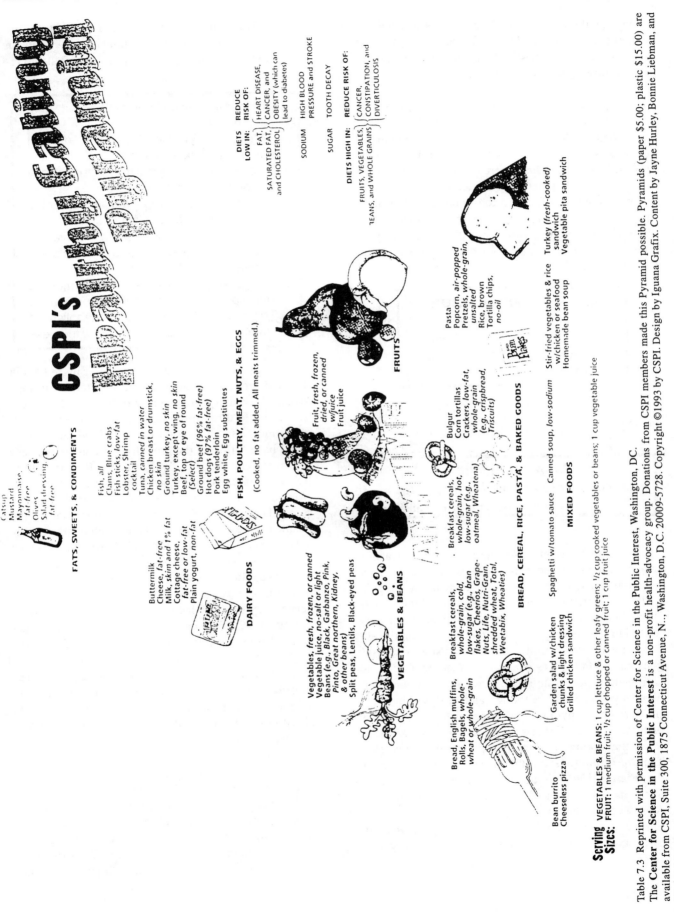

CSPI's Healthy Eating Pyramid

DIETS LOW IN:
- FAT, SATURATED FAT, and CHOLESTEROL } REDUCE RISK OF: HEART DISEASE, CANCER, and OBESITY (which can lead to diabetes)
- SODIUM — HIGH BLOOD PRESSURE and STROKE
- SUGAR — TOOTH DECAY

DIETS HIGH IN:
- FRUITS, VEGETABLES, BEANS, and WHOLE GRAINS } REDUCE RISK OF: CANCER, CONSTIPATION, and DIVERTICULOSIS

FATS, SWEETS, & CONDIMENTS

Catsup
Mustard
Mayonnaise, *fat-free*
Olives
Salad dressing, *fat-free*

FISH, POULTRY, MEAT, NUTS, & EGGS

(Cooked, no fat added. All meats trimmed.)

Fish, all
Clams, Blue crabs
Fish sticks, *low-fat*
Lobster, Shrimp cocktail
Tuna, *canned in water*
Chicken breast or drumstick, *no skin*
Ground turkey, *no skin*
Turkey, *except wing, no skin*
Beef, *top or eye of round (Select)*
Ground beef *(96% fat-free)*
Hot dogs *(97% fat-free)*
Pork tenderloin
Egg white, Egg substitutes

DAIRY FOODS

Buttermilk
Cheese, *fat-free*
Milk, *skim and 1% fat*
Cottage cheese, *fat-free or low-fat*
Plain yogurt, *non-fat*

FRUITS

Fruit, *fresh, frozen, dried, or canned w/juice*
Fruit juice

VEGETABLES & BEANS

Vegetables, *fresh, frozen, or canned*
Vegetable juice, *no-salt or light*
Beans *(e.g. Black, Garbanzo, Pink, Pinto, Great northern, Kidney, & other beans)*
Split peas, Lentils, Black-eyed peas

BREAD, CEREAL, RICE, PASTA, & BAKED GOODS

Bread, English muffins, Rolls, Bagels, *whole-wheat or whole-grain*
Breakfast cereals, *whole-grain, cold, low-sugar (e.g. bran flakes, Cheerios, Grape-Nuts, Life, Nutri-Grain, shredded wheat, Total, Weetabix, Wheaties)*
Breakfast cereals, *whole-grain, hot, low-sugar (e.g. oatmeal, Wheatena)*
Bulgur
Corn tortillas
Crackers, *low-fat, whole-grain (e.g. crispbread, Triscuits)*
Pasta
Popcorn, *air-popped*
Pretzels, *whole-grain, unsalted*
Rice, brown
Tortilla chips, *no-oil*

MIXED FOODS

Garden salad *w/chicken chunks & light dressing*
Grilled chicken sandwich
Spaghetti *w/tomato sauce*
Canned soup, *low-sodium*
Stir-fried vegetables & rice *w/chicken or seafood*
Homemade bean soup
Turkey *(fresh-cooked)* sandwich
Vegetable pita sandwich
Bean burrito
Cheeseless pizza

Serving Sizes: VEGETABLES & BEANS: 1 cup lettuce & other leafy greens; ½ cup cooked vegetables or beans; 1 cup vegetable juice
FRUIT: 1 medium fruit; ½ cup chopped or canned fruit; 1 cup fruit juice

Table 7.3 Reprinted with permission of Center for Science in the Public Interest, Washington, DC. Donations from CSPI members made this Pyramid possible. Pyramids (paper $5.00; plastic $15.00) are available from CSPI, Suite 300, 1875 Connecticut Avenue, N., Washington, D.C. 20009-5728. Copyright ©1993 by CSPI. Design by Iguana Grafix. Content by Jayne Hurley, Bonnie Liebman, and Michael Jacobson. The **Center for Science in the Public Interest** is a non-profit health-advocacy group.

as they regulate various body processes and help to maintain body tissue and bone. Refer to the *Nutrition Action Health Letter* listed at the end of this unit for more information about the use of supplements.

In the January 1994 issue of the *University of California at Berkeley Wellness Letter,* the editorial board changed their minds in regard to the recommendation of supplementary vitamins on a broad scale for healthy people. The research about the antioxidant vitamins E, C , A (plant form-betacarotene) plus the B vitamin, folacin, affects on the free radicals brought this change in thinking.   They state that *ideally* your vitamins should come from your diet but to protect yourself in the event that your diet is not supplying them you should supplement the above four.

DAILY RECOMMENDATIONS	
Vitamin E	None presently
Vitamin C	60 mg
Vitamin A	5,000 I.U.
Folic Acid	0.4 mg

Garlic

> *But for its odour -*
> *garlic would be costlier than gold.*
> ... Charak - father of Hindu medicine

This pleasant, but sometimes potent, seasoning ingredient has been in the news concerning its potential to help lower cholesterol, increase the blood's ability to clot, function as a natural antibiotic and strengthen the immune system. Research has been conducted in Europe, Japan and India for years on the effects of garlic on overall health. The history of garlic goes back 5,000 years where it is mentioned in Sanskrit manuscripts from India. It was also known to be used in China 3,000 years ago and in Egypt in 3750 B.C., when the pyramids were being built. It is also mentioned in the Hebrew book, the *Talmud,* where it states that taking garlic will help destroy "parasites." The *Old Testament* states that when journeying through the desert, sufficient rations of garlic went along. One of the most famous garlic stories is from the Middle Ages when the bubonic plague was on the rampage in Europe. It is reported that those who ate garlic in their diet survived at a ratio of three to one over non-garlic eaters.

This brings us to the question-What are the properties in garlic that bring about these effects on the body? The following have been identified and researched.

1. Allicin- has anti-inflammatory and anti-bacterial effects
2. Allithiamine (Vitamin B1)- helps prevent nervous and skin ailments
3. Selenium- helps prevent the build up of fatty placque in the blood vessels
4. Diallyldisulphide Oxide- this ingredient is what results when allicin is converted in the body and this is what is believed to lower the cholesterol and the lipids (fat substances) in the blood
5. Amino Acids- cystine and methionine which promote cellular growth and healing
6. Thiamine- helps with the metabolism of carbohydrates and also coping with stress

Garlic has been used as a major ingredient in the cuisine of India, China and the Mediterranean area. When I stayed at a yoga center in England I was told to eat two to three fresh whole cloves of garlic with every meal as it was good for my circulation. Since then I have followed the growth of interest in the beneficial effects of garlic . "A Promising Report on Garlic" was printed in the August, 1994 issue of *The Johns Hopkins Medical Letter: Health After 50.* A group of researchers at New York Medical College pooled the results of five studies that had appeared in major journals between 1987 and 1990. Their findings showed that a garlic supplement in powder, liquid or tablet form taken for 12-24 weeks in dosages of 600 to 1,000 mg daily (equivalent to two-thirds to one clove of garlic) resulted in a decreased cholesterol level by an average of 9%. They conclude with the suggestion that larger, better controlled studies are needed for a thorough understanding of the effects of garlic on cholesterol. The caution is made against too large of doses causing allergic reactions, flatulence, heartburn, drug interactions, unpleasant skin odor and a reduction in blood-clotting time. But there is no harm in using garlic as a seasoning.

Garlic is easy to grow and inexpensive to purchase. It is easy to develop the habit of cooking with garlic to enhance naturally your favorite recipes. Remember this New York Yiddish saying- "Three nickles will get you on the subway but **GARLIC** will get you a seat." To help overcome the after effects of eating raw garlic you can try one of the following remedies:

- Rinse mouth with 1/2 water and 1/2 lemon juice
- Chew on dill, fennel or anise seed
- Chew on roasted coffee ground and then spit out
- Eat a fresh apple
- Chew a slice of cinnamon or a whole clove
- Chew pieces of orange peel

In the spring of 1991 The First World Congress on the Health Significance of Garlic and Garlic Constitiuents was held in Washington, D.C. A group of over fifty medical experts and scientists met to discuss the modern discoveries about this ancient food. The reports showed that garlic and other alliums (onions, shallots) may erect a barrier against human cancer, increase the ability of the immune system's natural killer cells, and provide protection against heart and artery disease. Studies done in India showed lowered blood cholesterol, and in China and Japan they found garlic lowered blood-pressure. So Keep in mind the following-

> *Since garlic hath powers*
> *to save from death, bear with it*
> *though it makes unsavory breath.*
> **Salerno Regimine of Health- 12th century**

THREE APPROACHES TO EATING

Vegetarianism

Some people think that to properly "do yoga" you have to be a vegetarian or have no red-meat in your diet. This is not true. Yoga did develop in India, where people do not eat meat for a variety of reasons ranging from religious, and dietary choices, to economic and personal choices. There are several categories of a vegetarian diet.

- Traditional vegetarians: those whose eating habits have existed over generations due to a cultural belief and or lifestyle
- Total "vegans": no animal products at all are eaten
- Lacto-vegetarians: dairy products are eaten
- Lacto-ovo vegetarians: dairy products and eggs are eaten
- Semi-vegetarians: consume some groups of animal foods (no red meat but fish and chicken might be eaten)
- New vegetarians: developed after the 1960's, eat some form of a vegetarian diet along with foods that are considered to be less processed and more natural or organic

Many of the vegetarian diets are "millenia old and have stood the test of time with respect to the propagation of the species" as stated in the *Journal of American Dietetics Association* position paper on vegetarianism (1980- Vo. 77 p. 61-69).

A vegetarian diet is usually low in saturated fat and high in dietary fiber, which are highly recommended eating habits. Research studies done on Seventh-Day Adventists, who practice lacto-ovo and/or vegan eating habits, have shown that they have a lower mortality rate from coronary heart disease and cancer than the rest of our American population (see resources list at end of unit). There are several factors to consider when planning a vegetarian type diet, and they are as follows:

1. Select from a variety using the Food Guide Pyramid substituting the peas, beans and nuts for the meat group
2. Monitor the intake of the dairy group as you many need to increase the servings here.
3. Reduce (or eliminate) the empty calorie foods in your diet. (those that are high in calories and low in nutrients)
4. Increase the intake of complex carbohydrates (whole grain breads and cereals) to meet your energy requirements
5. Combine beans and wheat, beans and rice and lentils and rice, to get the amino acids from the protein that is necessary. Also eat *Quinoa (keen-wa),* which is a grain that has all the amino acids
6. If you are not consuming animal dairy products:
   a. drink fortified soybean milk
   b. provide Vitamin D as a supplement (check with physician)
   c. provide Vitamin B 12 as a supplement or eat foods high in B 12 (cereals, eggs, soy bean products made to resemble meat.) Read labels!

If you are curious about what a day's menu based on a vegetarian diet is like refer to Table 7.4 for a sample menu of a lacto-ovo vegetarian diet.

Sample Menus for Lacto-ovo Vegetarian Diet

Meal and Food Group	Menu 1	Menu 2
Breakfast		
Milk	Milk	Milk
Meat Alternate		Scrambled egg or tofu (soy curd)
Fruit-Vegetable	Orange	Prune juice
Grain	Oatmeal	Shredded wheat
	Date-nut muffin	Wheat soy bread
Others	Butter/margarine	Butter/margarine
	Coffee/hot cereal	Coffee/hot cereal
Lunch		
Milk	Cream Mushroom Soup (made with milk)	Cottage Cheese for Fruit Plate
Meat Alternate	Peanut Butter for Sandwich	Lentil Soup
Ruit-Vegetable	Carrot Sticks	Apricots, Grapefruit
	Banana	Pineapple, Grapes, Lettuce Leaves in Fruit Plate
Grain	Rye Crackers	Whole Wheat Crackers
	Whole Wheat Bread	
Others	Beverage	Salad Dressing
		Beverage
Dinner		
Milk	Yogurt	
Meat Alternate	Baked Beans	Quiche - milk, egg
Fruit-Vegetable	Corn	Broccoli
	Collards	Spinach Salad
	Sliced Tomato Salad	
Grain	Brown Bread	Whole Wheat Roll
Others	Salad Dressing	Salad Dressing
	Butter/Margarine	Butter/Margarine
	Tea/Hot Cereal	Tea/Hot Cereal
	Beverage	Beverage
Snacks		
	Cheese	Sunflower Seeds
	Crackers	Apple

Vegetarian Nutrition. National Dairy Council. 1979, Rosemont, IL 60018

Table 7.4 *Vegetarian Diet*

ANTI-CANCER DIET

Research in epidemiology has discovered some connections between dietary habits, dietary intake, and cancer. It has been discovered that the following nutrients may have a positive impact on lowering the risk of cancer:

1. <u>Cruciferous Vegetables</u> - broccoli, brussel sprouts, cabbage, cauliflower, bok choy, collord greens,kale, kohlrabi, mustard and turnip greens, rutabagas and turnips
2. <u>Beta Carotene</u> - converts to Vitamin A in the body -carrots, apricots, cantaloupe, papayas, nectarines, watermelon, broccoli, sweet potatoes, winter squash and all dark leafy vegetables
3. <u>Vitamin C</u> - helps with cellular strengthening -primarialy citrus fruits
4. <u>Vitamin E</u> - peppers, spinach, carrots, broccoli, rice, wheat and oats, yeast and vegetable oils, and liver
5. <u>Fiber</u> - whole grains and fresh fruits and vegetables

The American Institute for Cancer Reserch (AICR) has a newsletter and numerous pamphlets that are helpful when learning how to lower cancer risk. They have outlined recommendations which are similar to the guidelines from the United States Government and the Center for Science in the Public Interest. These AICR suggestions resulted from the work of nutritionist Jerry Rivers Ph. D. and Karen Collins, M.S., R. D.

1. Reduce the intake of dietary fat- both saturated and unsaturated
2. Increase the consumption of fruits, vegetables and whole grain cereals
3. Consume salt-cured, smoked and charcoal-broiled foods only in moderation
4. Drink alcoholic beverages only in moderation

The National Cancer Institute has been studying the chemical components of the edible plants in the cancer protective foods recommended for our consumption. The substances looked at are called *phytochemicals* - and Herbert Pierson, a toxicologist, has been studying them since 1989. He has been focusing his research on garlic, flaxseed, citrus fruits, licorice root, parsley, carrots and celery. When asked in the article in the *Nutrition Action Health Letter,* (April 1991) "Can you tell us now which foods prevent cancer?" Pierson replied "Recommendations have to come from the National Cancer Institute. I can say that it won't hurt to eat more garlic, to keep your diet varied, and to eat as many fruits, vegetables and whole grains as you can tolerate" (p. 7).

You may now want to refer to a sample menu from AICR ,Table 7.5, which is based upon the above recommendations. The recipes will be in the recipe section in the appendix.

Menu Using all Food Groups

Breakfast
1/4 cup Ready-to Eat Whole Grain Cereal
1/2 cup Cantaloupe
1/2 cup Lowfat Milk
1 1/2 cup Skim or Lowfat Milk

Salad Bar Lunch
Salad Bar with Small Wedge Lettuce
1/2 cup Carrot
1/4 cup Raw Cauliflower
1/2 cup Garbanzo or Kidney Beans
2 Tbsp. Regular Salad Dressing
6 Whole Grain Rye Wafers

Quick-to-Fix Dinner
6 oz. chicken (or Veal) Piccata (pounded very thin, cooked quickly and flavored with lemon and parsley)
1 cup Whole Wheat Noodles with 1 1/2 tsp. Margarine
1/4 cup Tomato-Basil Salad

Evening Snack
1 Bran Muffin

Table 7.5   *Anti-Cancer Eating Plan*

Longevity Diet

A diet that is "high" in nutrient quality and "low" in calories is recommended by Roy L. Walford, M.D., a professor of Pathology at the University of California at Los Angeles and one of this country's leading researchers in the field of aging and life extension. He recommends that we "increase the ratio of fish to red meat in the diet, increase vegetable protein in relation to animal protein (this will lower the amount of fat in the diet), increase the amount of complex carbohydrates, cut back sharply on refined sugars, and make sure that copper and chromium intake are not greatly below the Recommended Daily Allowance levels" (Walford, p 124).He also suggest that you raise your magnesium intake over the current average amount, let the ratio of magnesium/calcium in your diet be 1.1 and increase the intake of gel-forming fibers such as bran. He recommends adequate calcium and lower amounts of fat and sodium to help protect the body from disease. Dr. Walford's book, *The 120-Year Diet* , discusses in great detail the impact of good nutritional practices on the body. It presents 20 days of computer-generated, nutrient-dense, low-calorie menus with recipes, as well as a chart of the nutritive values of the best foods. This book is full of sound nutritional advice (see resources).

WEIGHT MANAGEMENT

> *In reality, a very overweight person*
> *should perform light exercise*
> *for long periods of time.*
> *This is the only way the metabolism of*
> *such an individual will begin to burn fat.*
> *. . .* **Deepak Chopra, M.D.**

Dean Ornish, M.D., who has conducted research with heart disease patients placed his subjects on a total vegetarian diet. Along with the heart disease reversal that is discussed in Unit 9, he found that during the first year, the patients in the Lifestyle Heart Trial lost an average of 22 pounds. This was done without counting calories, without measuring portion sizes, without hunger all while they were eating more frequently and were eating more food. They were not eating fat calories. On this eating plan the participants could eat any of the folllowing foods whenever they were hungry: beans and legumes, fruits, grains, vegetables. They could eat in moderation: nonfat dairy products and egg whites, and nonfat or very low-fat commercially available products. The food items "to avoid as much as possible" were: meats (all kinds including chicken and fish), oils (all kinds), avocados, olives, nuts and seeds, dairy products including high-fat or low-fat, sugar, alcohol and any commercial product with more than two grams of fat. " That is all there is to it," reports Dr. Ornish (*Yoga Journal* Nov./Dec. 1993). His book, *Eat More, Weigh Less,* has an abundance of delicious low-fat, no-fat vegetarian recipes.

One of the main discoveries in regard to weight management has come from the National Institute of Health Center's "respiratory chamber" in Phoenix, Arizona. People come to this chamber at a motel and spend 24 hours while they are being monitored by sensors that will calculate their every move and the calories burned or not burned. The researchers are able to determine if the calories burned have come from carbohydrates or fat. As a result the researchers are able to discover the clients metabolism level and how weight is gained. Some people's bodies do not burn fat and once they know this they then realize that "**fat**" is something they can not ingest. The storage of carbohydrates in the body is carefully regulated by the body but the storage of fat is not. Limited amounts of excess carbohydrates are stored as glycogen in the liver. Fat is stored all over the body in the fat cells that are already there.

Researchers from the Howard Hughes Medical Institute at Rockefeller University in New York announced that they had located in mice the gene that caused obesity and also found that the new gene called "obese" very likely exists in humans. They have discovered that this "ob gene" can direct cells to produce a protein also known as "ob." This protein seems to be the chemical that tells the mice they are satieted and to stop eating. In the "ob/ob mice" this protein is broken and the brain doesn't get the signal to quit eating. With the discovery of this gene scientists can now trace the link between the gene and the resulting obesity.

The Dana-Farber Cancer Institute, in the journal *Cell,* reported the discovery of another protein that converts cells into fat cells in very overweight people. Even, with all of this recent research the best approach to managing weight is to exercise and lead an active lifestyle with a sensible, low-fat/no-fat eating plan.

OVERWEIGHT

When beginning to do yoga people usually develop a greater appreciation for their physical self and thus want to take better care of themself. This can lead to changes in eating and exercise habits. Hatha yoga with its gentle approach, can be done by those who are overweight

Two women, Genia Pauli Haddon and Linda DeMarco, both with a plump body build, collaborated on a three-hour at home yoga video, *Yoga for Round Bodies.* These videos were developed from their own personal experience of having rounded bodies and knowing what yoga poses they could do comfortably , and also how to adapt the asanas for their bodies. They emphasize an " attitude of non-critical self observation. Let your intention be to discover how each posture lives within your own unique body." (*Yoga Journal,* Sept/Oct. 1994 p. 90). They also recommend the use of props to assist with proper alignment.

Most of the yoga poses in this book can be done safely by people who are under 20-25 pounds overweight. If you are over your desirable weight by 25 pounds, then refer to the following precautions.

Precautions

1. Inverted poses done with caution:
   a. Headstand hang, headstand and the handstand poses should not be done when alone and only with an experienced teacher
   b. Shoulderstand by the wall
   c. Dolphin for a short time and then repeat 2 times

SUMMARY

"A Journey of a Thousand miles begins with ONE step"
... Lao Tsze

There is much information in this unit which may have overwhelmed you. To help you sort through all of this I will attempt to pull it all together with some basic suggestions that have appeared throughout and add a few more.

1. Eating should be pleasurable, but not the central focus of your life. Think of food as providing the fuel, and necessary ingredients to keep your body running for a long and healthy life.
2. Remember this basic idea using the yoga approach- Try to eat foods as close to their natural state as your digestion permits
3. Make changes in your diet gradually
4. Read food labels
5. Keep your nutrient and fiber content HIGH
6. Keep the amount of fat and fried foods, overprocessed food ingested LOW
7. Make wise decisions at "fast food eating places"
8. Keep your total caloric intake at the level desirable for you
9. Assess your nutritional intake to see if you need vitamin and mineral supplements. Vegetarians may need to supplement with Vitamin B12
10. Daily eat: from all of the food groups, some of the anti-cancer food and a little garlic!

Now have some fun trying out some of the recipes that are in Appendix F.

RESOURCES

Books

Bailey, Covert and Bishop, Lea. *The Fit or Fat Woman.* Boston MA: Houghton Mifflin Company, 1989.

Balch, James F. M.D. and Phyllis A. Balch, C.N.C. *Prescription for Nutritional Healing.* Garden City Park, New York: Avery Publishing Group Inc., 1990.

Brody, Jane. *Jane Brody's Nutrition Book.* New York, N.Y.: W.W. Norton & Co., 1981.

Chopra, Deepak, M.D. *Perfect Weight.* New York: Harmony Books, 1994.

Gilroy, People of. *The Complete Garlic Lovers' Cookbook.* Berkeley. CA: Celestial Arts, 1987.

Hausman, Patricia and Judith Benn Hurley. *The Healing Foods,* Emmaus, PA. Rodale Press, 1989.

Klaper, Michael M.D., *Vegan Nutrition; Pure and Simple,* Alachua, Fl: Gentle World Publishing, 1987

Lappe, Frances Moore. *Diet for A Small Planet,* New York: Ballantine Books, 1982.

Madison, Deborah and Brown, Edward E. *The Greens Cook Book* New York, NY: Bantam. 1987.

Ornish, Dean M.D. *Eat More, Weigh Less,* New York: Harper Collins Publishers, 1993.

Robertson, Laurel. et al. *Laurel's Kitchen,* Berkeley, CA: Ten Speed Press, 1993.

Walford, Roy MD. *The 120 Year Diet.* New York: Simon and Schuster, 1986.

_____*Anti-Aging Diet.* New York, NY Four Walls Eight Windows Publishing, 1994

Wood, Rebecca. *Quinoa, The Supergrain: Ancient Food for Today.* Tokyo, Japan: Japan Publications, Inc. 1989. (US distributor, New York, Harper & Row)

Publications

Haddon, Genia Pauli, "Yoga for Round Bodies," *Yoga Journal,* Sept./Oct. 1994 p. 88-97.

Hurley, Jayne and Stephen Schmidt. "A Clove a Day?," *Nutrition Action Healthletter.* December, 1989, p.8-9.

" A Promising Report on Garlic," *The Johns Hopkins Medical Letter: Health After 50.* August 1994, p.1.

Jaret, Peter. "Eating Your Crucifers Really Can Cut Your Chances of Getting Cancer," *In HEALTH.* Sept/Oct. 1991, p. 59-61, 62.

"The Way to Lose Weight," *In Health,* Jan./Feb. 1995. p. 52-58.

Liebman, Bonnie. "Getting Your Vitamins?" *Nutrition Action Healthletter.* June 1990. p.1, 5-7.

"Designer Foods", *Nutrition Action Health Letter.* April 1991, p.1, 5-7.

Schardt, David. "Phytochemicals: Plants Against Cancer," *Nutrition Action Health Letter.* April 1994 p.1,9-11.

"Making the Most of Fast Food Meals". *American Institute for Cancer Research Newsletter.* Summer 1990. p. 6

Wirkner, Linda. "A Healthy Flavor," *Key Horizons.* Spring 1992. p. 50-52, 54-56.

Magazines To Subscribe To

American Institute for Cancer Research Newsletter. Published by the American Institute for Cancer Research. 1759 R. Street N.W. Washington, D.C. 20009, (202) 328-7744.

Nutrition Action Health Letter. Published by the Center for Science in the Public Interest. 1875 Conneticut Ave NW Suite 300, Washington, D. C. 20009-5728

Tufts University Diet & Nutrition Letter. For subscription: Box 57857, Boulder, Co. 80322.

Veggie Life. EGW Publishing Co., 1041 Shary Circle, Concord Ca. 94518.

Vegetarian Times. P.O. Box 5042, Clifton, NJ 07015.

Video

Yoga for Round Bodies, Linda deMarco and Genia Pauli Haddon. Plus Publications 800-793-0666.

Yoga for Special Populations

> *May all be happy, May all be free from disease,*
> *May all look to the good of others,*
> *May none suffer from sorrow.*
>   **. . . Anonymous**

Yoga has been recommended as an exercise program for people who have a need for some type of adaptation. Yoga lends itself to adaptions very readily. Yoga has also been used as a form of therapy for common problems such as headaches, constipation, back problems or a lack of flexibility. Mr. B.K.S. Iyengar's book *Light on Yoga* , has a section where all forms of health conditions are listed with the appropriate yoga asana that can possibly help with the condition. Unit 9 will discuss further the therapeutic use of yoga.

In this section some of the most common concerns and adaptations will be discussed. Topics covered will be menstrual disorders, pregnancy, yoga for children/young people and older adults, wheelchair yoga, and yoga for the visually impaired. The asanas that are especially helpful will be listed. What should not be done will be mentioned as well as modifications of the traditional poses when it is feasible. You can refer to the chart, Table 8.1, for a handy reference to locate the poses that should NOT be done or are to be done with caution.

MENSTRUAL DISORDERS

Judith Lasater, P.T. and Ph.D., recommends for premenstrual syndrom (PMS) that women do the shoulderstand and the forward bending and twisting poses.

Special Conditions and Yoga Asanas

Code: * Avoid doing   ▲ Do With Caution

	Breath (Hold)	Shoulder-stand	Dog	Hang Head-Stand	Dolphin	Chest Expansion	Bow	Full Locust	Cobra	Plough
Menstrual Cramps		*		*						
Pregnant	*	*	▲	*			*	*	*	*
High Blood Pressure	*	▲		*	▲	▲		*		
Eye Concern	▲	▲	▲	*	▲	▲		▲		
Neck		▲		*			▲	▲	*	
Low Back							▲	▲	▲	*
Scoliosis				▲						
Obese		*		*				▲		*

Table 8.1

Precautions:

1. The inverted pose of the shoulderstand, headstand hang and headstand are not to be done DURING the menstrual cycle.

Recommended Asanas
for Menstrual Disorders:

```
Cat  (Fig. 3.21A,B & C)
Spinal Twist (Fig. 8.7A & B)
Arrow Sit (Fig 4.7)
Sitting Forward Bend (Fig. 3.18A&B)
Dog ( Fig. 3.23)
Back Pushup (Fig. 3.22)
* Headstand (Fig. 4.6)
* Shoulderstand (Fig. 3.25 A-E)
Fish  (Fig. 3.26)

* Do not do during menstrual cycle.
```

PREGNANCY

There is much more information available for the pregnant woman who wants to continue to exercise now than there was a few years ago. The American College of Obstetrics and Gynecologists have a 1994 position paper "Exercise During Pregnancy and the Postpartum Period," Technical Bulletin #189, February, that is available. It is recommended that you always check with your physician before beginning an exercise program. If you have been doing hatha yoga and your pregnancy is progressing normally, it is fine to continue. The gentle approach of yoga and the use of the breath makes it an ideal form of exercise during pregnancy. It can improve your circulation and keep your muscles pliant and can even help make the delivery easier. Always remember to do the relaxation and complete breath daily as this will assist you during delivery. Try to maintain an erect standing posture to protect the muscles of the low back. During pregnancy the breasts become larger to prepare for breastfeeding thus the pectoral muscles underneath the breasts should be strengthened.

Dr. Mary Pullig Schatz, in her *Back Care Basics,* book makes the following recommendation for sleeping and exercising during pregnancy; " When you are lying on your back, the enlarging uterus can compress the vena cava (the huge vein at the back of the pelvis that drains the legs, pelvis, and abdomen, re-turning the blood to the heart). For this reason, avoid lying on your back during the second half of pregnancy." Use a pillow and folded blankets to support your abdomen and legs when lying on your side (Schatz. p. 191).

Precautions:

1. When doing your pranayama, do not hold the breath. Keep the breath flowing in and out.
2. Do NOT do the inverted poses, headstand hang, headstand or shoulderstand as there is the possibility of placing the fetus next to the top part of the uterus where it may be attached to the placenta. This could place too much pressure at this site.
3. Once the abdomen is becoming large do not do the asanas requiring you to lie on your abdomen. You will know when as it will no longer feel comfortable or "right" for you.

Recommendation:

1. Practice the deep breathing daily.
2. In the early stages, do the abdominal toning exercises or yoga sitback and up and the single abdominal lift.
3. Elevate your legs by the wall following the directions in unit 3 (Fig 8.6).
4. Check yourself in the mountain pose in front of a mirror every week to monitor your postural alignment.
5. Do a standing balance asana daily. As your abdomen increases your sense of balance and center of gravity are changing. Daily practice should help you stay more centered as well as strengthen the feet and legs. Practice by a chair or wall for support.
6. Practice sitting in a squat position. Again use a chair, wall or pillow to stabilize yourself if you want (Fig 8.1A & B).
7. Practice sitting in a wide straddle position (Fig. 8.3).
8. Post Pregnancy: When you have the approval of your physician, begin strengthening your abdominal muscles. If a cesearean section has been done you will need to be more cautious. The pelvic tilt, cat, and yoga sit back are good ones to begin with as well as the single abdominal lift. You must put effort into strengthening these muscles as soon as you can
9. Check the resources section for books and videos for yoga during pregnancy and for relaxation music for infants.

Recommended Asanas
for Pregnancy:

Mountain Pose (Fig. 3.13)
Tree (Fig. 3.28)
Chest Expansion (Fig. 3.20)
Squatting (Fig. 8.1A &B)
Back Stretch at wall or ballet barre(3.7)
Alternate Leg Stretch (Fig. 3.12)
Knee Thigh Stretch (Fig.8.2)
Straddle Sitting (Fig. 8.3)
Cat (Fig. 8.4)
Dog (Fig. 8.5)
Warrior II on Chair(Fig 4.15b)
Spinal Twist in chair (Fig. 8.7A &B)
Legs elevated by Wall(Fig. 8.6)

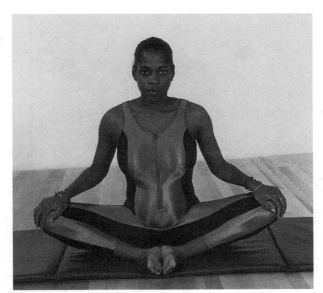

Figure 8.2   *Knee Thigh Stretch*

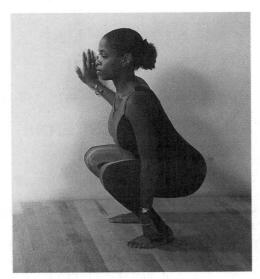

Figure 8.1A   *Squatting*

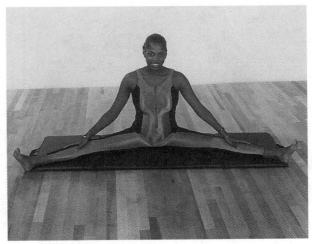

Figure 8.3   *Straddle Sitting*

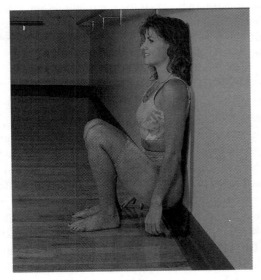

Figure 8.1B   *Squatting*

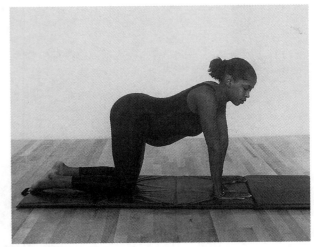

Figure 8.4A   *Cat*

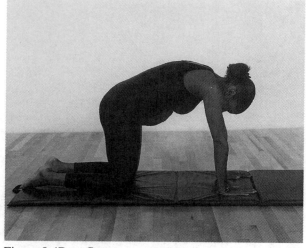

Figure 8.4B   *Cat*

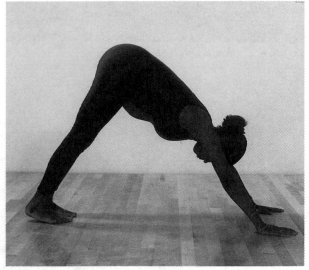

Figure 8.5   *Dog*

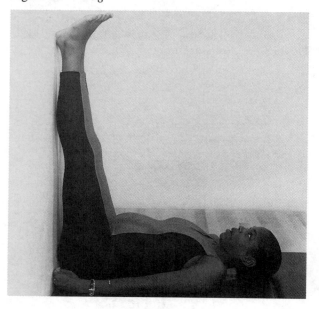

Figure 8.6   *Legs Elevated by Wall*

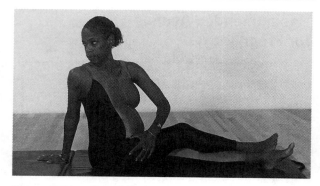

Figure 8.7A   *Spinal Twist*

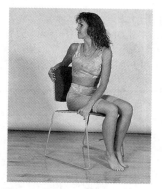

Figure 8.7B   *Spinal Twist in Chair*

VISUAL CONCERNS

Yoga is an ideal activity for those with vision problems. As the teacher, the basic guideline to remember is to give precise verbal cues and directions and leave nothing to the imagination. I thank each one of the visually impaired students I have had in yoga as they <u>taught</u> me a lot about teaching the asanas to them. The environment in which yoga is taught is a safe one for a blind person. They can feel comfortable as there is less movement among the class members. Also, the use of partners contributes to the sense of being in a safe environment. Many poses are done on the floor thus there is less risk of falling.

The benefits are many. The visualization cues can help with the body image. As they gain in awareness of how they can move their body there is a gain in self confidence. The mobility is enhanced and they gain a greater sense of balance due to the practice of the balance asanas. What is taught as yoga poses, such as Tadasana, can be applied to their basic posture and movement in their daily life. There can be tension in the neck and back muscles from walking in a protective posture. The reduction of stress and the benefits gained from the breathing and the relaxation are the same as for those who are sighted. As shown in Fig. 8.8, a visually impaired student and her guide dog can do Hatha Yoga together.

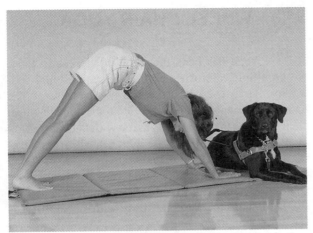

Figure 8.8 *Visually Impaired Student with Guide Dog*

Precautions

1. If the vision problem (such as glaucoma or retina damage) could be worsened by bringing blood to the head do NOT do the inverted poses of dog, headstand hang, or headstand and do chest expansion for 5-10 seconds only.

Recommendations

1. If the directions for doing the poses are not clear ask a teacher to help you.
2. Use a small, wooden mannequin that is jointed and place in the asana. The student can then feel with the hands the shape and with this " image" through touching can then do the pose.

YOGA EYE EXERCISES

The eyes are moved by muscles,therefore they too can benefit from exercise. Relaxing exercises for the eyes are included in the practice of yoga from India, and acupuncture and acupressure from China. The yoga eye exercises involve movement, while the acupressure approach is through massage. All of these exercises increase the circulation to the eye muscles and can help relieve eyestrain and that tired feeling we have from time spent at the computer or reading. Doing these exercises while wearing contacts or glasses is all right but you may prefer to remove them.

Two types of eye exercises will be taught - the hatha yoga eye exercises and the Chinese eye exercises.. Following are the basic directions. Seat yourself comfortably. Do not move the head; move <u>only the eyes.</u> Keep breathing normally and allow the rest of your body to become fully relaxed. These exercises are simple to do and can be done at almost any time or place.

HATHA YOGA EYE EXERCISES

Tracking to the Right and Left
1. Gazing straight in front of you, find a spot to be your center focal point.
2. Slowly and smoothly move the eyes to the right as far as they can go; now move them to the left as far as they can go. Repeat.
3. Blink your eyes, then close them to rest.

Tracking Up and Down
1. Gazing straight in front of you, find a spot to be your center focal point.
2. Slowly and smoothly move the eyes up as far as they will go. (you can probably see the fringe of your hair). Now slowly and smoothly move them down (now you can probably see the side of your nose). Repeat.
3. Blink your eyes, then close them and allow them to rest.

Clock Tracking
1. Gazing straight in front of you, find a spot to be your center focal point; this is where the imaginary hands of the clock are attached.
2. Now, slowly and smoothly move your eyes up to 12 o'clock, then slowly around to 1 and 2 o'clock. At 3 o'clock, the eyes should be as far to the right as they can go. Then move on to 4 and 5. At 6 o'clock the eyes are looking down. Continue on to 7 and 8. At 9 o'clock the eyes are over to the far left. Move on to 10, ll, and finally 12 o'clock, at which time you are gazing up as far as your eyes can go. Now reverse the movement, moving the eyes to 11, 10, 9 o'clock, etc.
3. Finish by closing your eyes. Place your palms over them and allow them a few minutes to rest.

As you did these exercises, did you notice a feeling of warmth around the eyes? Did they water? These are common responses because the eyes are probably not used to doing these exercises. Exercising the eyes will not necessarily correct any eye problems, but it is a way of strengthening the muscles and improving circulation. Once you try them you will find they are very refreshing and relaxing and should be done periodically while you are studying.

CHINESE EYE EXERCISES

These exercises involve a massaging action which is stimulating therefore increasing the circulation to the eyes. The sinuses may also respond. You will notice this by the urge to sniff or blow your nose. An art student from China taught these exercises to one of our yoga classes and told us that children from pre-school age through teenage years do them during their school day.

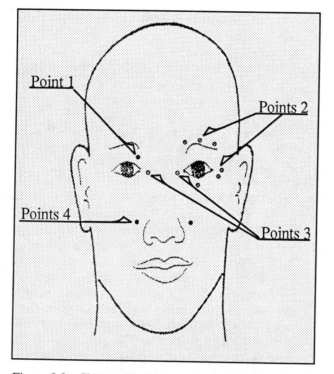

Figure 8.9 *Chinese Eye Exercise Placement of Hands*

1. Place thumbs in the inner corner of the eye on the boney area. Find a slight depression and press and move the thumbs in circles. Elbows are directed forward. Do 8 circular motions and then reverse direction and repeat.
2. The thumbs are on the temples. The index fingers are bent and massage across the bone on the eyebrow and below the eye opening of the skull. Do 8 wipes above and 8 below the eye.
3. Place the thumb and the finger on the bridge of the nose by the tear ducts and pull up pinching slightly 4 times. Do 4 more with the other hand.
4. Place the index fingers by the cheek bones in a depression near the nostrils of the nose and make 8 circular motions and reverse the direction for 8 more.

WHEEL CHAIR YOGA

Yoga has been taught with success to those with multiple sclerosis, cerebral palsy, muscular dystrophy, Parkinson's disease and heart disease. The hatha yoga asanas can be modified to be done in wheel chairs. Using the neckties to assist with the body alignment is also helpful for those with a disability. Learning to use the breath to calm and to energize the body is also of great benefit for those who are disabled in some way. The benefits of relaxation, music and visualization are the same for those with a disability as for those who have none.

At Ickwell Bury, England, there is a residential center run by the Yoga for Health Foundation under the direction of Howard Kent. Here, those with a disability can come and stay for any length of time and be supervised in doing yoga, learn pranayama, meditation, and enjoy eating nutritious meals. The staff consists of yoga teachers, a nurse, a physical therapist, a massage therapist and a physician who makes "house calls" and is available for consulting. Seminars and training programs in remedial yoga and medical problems are also sponsored by the center. You can find the address in the resources section.

For more information and for first hand accounts of yoga helping those with a disability you can refer to the books and articles listed in the resources section.

Recommendations

1. If possible do the yoga poses on a mat.
2. If staying in the chair lean away from the back so you are able to better use the muscles of your abdomen and back in the asanas to strengthen them.
3. Take the responsibility for your daily practice of yoga and deep breathing.

RECOMMENDED ASANAS FOR THOSE IN WHEELCHAIRS:

SITTING
1. Neck stretches (Fig. 3.1)
2. Neck turns (Fig. 3.2)
3. Chest expansion (Fig. 3.20)
4. Head of the Cow (Fig. 3.19 & 10.6)
5. Eye exercises (above)
6. Lion (Fig. 3.33)
7. Single and Both knees to chest in chair or on the mat (Fig. 3.4, 3.5 &3.17)
8. Abdominal lift (Fig. 3.31)
9. Alternate leg stretch with necktie in chair or on mat (Fig. 3.12)
10. Spinal Twist in chair or on mat (Fig. 8.7A&B)
11. Triangle (Fig. 3.29) - sitting it becomes a side bend
12. Triangle Twist (Fig. 3.30)- sitting placing the opposite hand on the opposite leg or chair arm
13. Try these routines:
    a. Moon Salute
    b. A sitting "Sun Salute" was developed and printed in the *Yoga Journal* (see resource)

ON A FLOOR MAT
1. Cobra (Fig. 3.14A & 3.14B)
2. Shoulderstand (Fig. 3.25A & B) - with the legs at the wall do some foot circles and flex and point each foot
3. Fish pose (Fig. 3.26) - may need assistance to lift into arch
4. Yoga sit back and if strong enough do the Yoga sit back AND UP (Fig. 3.24)
5. Fetus (Fig.3.16A &B)
6. Feldenkrais kneeovers (Fig. 3.10)
7. Crocodile Routine of Swami Dev Murti, Unit

YOGA FOR YOUNG PEOPLE

One of my career goals has been to assist in bridging the gap between the practice of yoga and the physical education profession. As a physical education undergraduate student at the University of Nebraska, I discovered Hatha Yoga and was impressed with all that it had to offer in the way of becoming fit and strong. The fact that it is an activity that can be continued throughout ones life time also appealed to me. My first teaching of Hatha Yoga was to high school girls physical education classes in 1966-70, and they loved it. Consequently, I have continued to teach and to do presentations at national and international conferences in hopes that more physical education teachers will include Hatha Yoga in their curriculum.

Children enjoy doing yoga. The concept of "baby yoga" with the photos of the early movement patterns of infants, was presented in unit 2, Yoga Basics. Hatha yoga poses mimic the movement of animals which is easy for children to relate to . The fact that this is a gentle and noncompetitive form of exercise is appealing to many parents as well as children. The style of improving strength, flexibility, and teaching children to concentrate, relax, and how to use their breath can be carried over into their life and other activities- the same as for an adult.

A very helpful book was written by a special education college professor who was also a yoga student/ teacher, for parents of children who are "distracted". She had discovered the personal benefits of yoga and realized that the practice of yoga would probably also benefit children who were having learning and concentration difficulties. Her approach focused on the use of imagery, relaxation, deep breathing, control of the senses, and internal scanning when doing the yoga poses (Burford. *How to Focus the Distractible Child.*) . See the resources.

The teen years can be a very stressful time for young people. Working with the physical self doing Hatha Yoga aids in building self esteem and a healthy body image. Since yoga is an individualized activity without competition young people can learn to value themselves the way they are and learn to do activities that improve their posture, balance and graceful movement, and lower their stress. One of the other positive aspect of doing yoga is that it is an activity that young people and their parents can do together both benefitting and reenforcing the good habit of exercise.

Yoga Session for Young People

Butterfly-Knee Thigh Stretch (Fig. 3.4)
Tree (Fig. 8.15, .16, .17)
Triangle (Fig. 3.29)
Lion (Fig. 3.33)
Cobra (Fig. 8.10)
Cat (Fig. 8.11)
Squats (Fig. 8.12)
Dog (Fig. 8.13)
Plank (Fig. 8.14)
Half Locust (Fig. 3.15)
Folded Leaf (Fig. 3.16B)
Relax, Complete Breath (Fig. 6.1)

Yoga for Young People

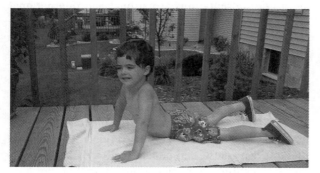

Figure 8.10   *Cobra*

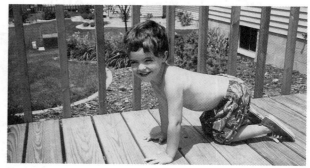

Figure 8.11   *Cat*

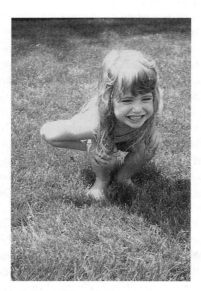

Figure 8.12   *Squats*

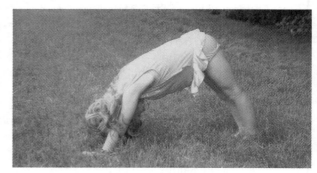

Figure 8.13   *Dog*

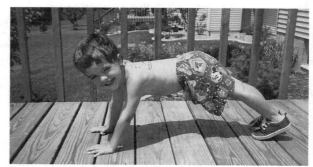

Figure 8.14   *Plank*

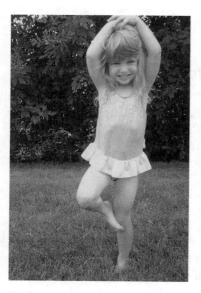

Figure 8.15   *Tree*

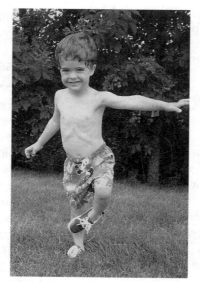

Figure 8.16   *Tree*

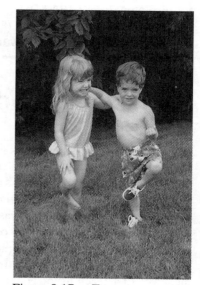

Figure 8.17   *Tree*

YOGA FOR OLDER ADULTS

> *At my age, I thought that I was just too old for Yoga...This yoga is nice and easy and that's why I like it so much.*
>
> **Mae Norris, 84 years.** *Easy Does It Yoga, p.32.*

I became aware of the merits of yoga for older adults when I first began teaching hatha yoga to the Elderhostelers who came to Ball State University. I taught one week sessions of 1 1/2 hour classes for several summers. Even in only one week the benefits were apparent. One gentleman, who after the third day, practiced the complete breath in the relaxation position when going to sleep. The result was the most restful sleep he had experienced since he had been plagued with bursitis in his shoulder. The breathing control, the relaxation, stress reduction, and balance asanas as well as all of the poses that improve flexibility, muscular strength and posture are a natural for older persons to learn.

There is no better example of yoga being practiced in later years than the story of the now famous "Delany Sisters" of Mt. Vernon, NY. At the time they wrote their book *Having Our Say; The Delany Sisters' First 100 Years,* Sadie was 103 and Bessie was 101. Sadie had started doing yoga exercises with their mother about forty years previous- when she was about 60 years old. She continued on another 20 years after her mother died . When Bessie turned eighty she " . . . decided that I (Sadie) looked better than her. So she decided she would start doing yoga, too.. So we've been doing our exercises together ever since. We follow a yoga exercise program on the TV." Photographs of them in the yoga poses of the shoulderstand, the spinal twist and the foot behind the head have been shown in magazines. They also eat a clove of garlic after their yoga practice, eat as many as seven different vegetables a day plus lots of fresh fruits. They also take vitamin supplements and ever since moving to their house in 1957 they have boiled their tap water and grow and can alot of their own vegetables. When asked about the key to living a long, fulfilling life, their answer was "Discipline. If you're young," Sadie says, "that means working or studying hard. When you're our age, it means exercising every day, whether you feel like it or not." (*The Delany Sisters' Book of Everyday Wisdom, 1994).* What an inspiration these two delightful energetic women are.*

*Bessie Delaney died at home in her sleep, Sept. 25, 1995.

The following yoga recommendations were developed for my book, *Forever Fit: A Step by Step Guide for Older Adults,* that I wrote with my sister-in-law Susan Birkel Freitag. An older person should consult with their physician before they begin a hatha yoga class and should share with the teacher their health history and the physicians recommendations. A form for this purpose was developed by me and a committee of exercise physiologists and medical doctors: the *Medical/Exercise Assessment Form.* This form is available from The American Alliance of Health, Physical Education, Recreation and Dance sub group, the Council on Aging and Adult Development.

As the teacher, you should be familiar with all of the precautions for the poses and pass that information on to the older adults. Especially emphasize:

1. Do **not** hold the breath in the poses if a person has elevated blood pressure or other symptoms of heart disease
2. Do **not** leave the arms over the head for very long (eg. mountain pose).
3. Do **not** leave the head lower than the heart if a person has elevated blood pressure, glaucoma or retina problems. (eg. dog, standing forward bend, and the inverted poses)

The following is a series of asanas that are of benefit to the older adult and can be safely done following the above recommendations.

Older Adult Hatha Yoga Routine

SITTING:
Yoga Complete Breath (page 75)
Head Turns (Fig. 3.1)
Toe Hold Leg Lift with Tie (Fig. 3.11B)
Foot Circles

STANDING:
Tree (Fig. 3.28)
Abdominal Lift (Fig. 3.31)
Chest Expansion (Fig. 3.20)
Head of Cow (Fig. 3.19)

ON FLOOR:
Cobra (Fig. 3.14A)
Cat (Fig. 3.21A, B, & C)
Dog (Fig. 3.23)
Back Push-Up (Fig. 8.18)
Shoulderstand or Feet and Legs Elevated at Wall   (Fig. 3.25 & 8.6)
Fish (Fig. 8.19)
Knees to Chest (Fig. 3.17)
Relax

Also recommended are the Moon Salute Routine (Fig. 3.35) and the Crocodile Routine (Fig. 6.4)

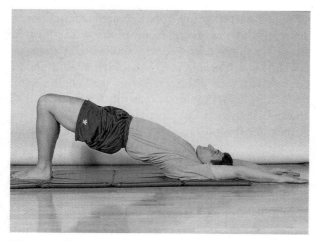

Figure 8.18   *Back Push-Up*

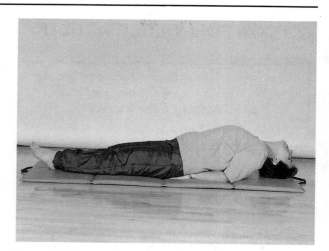

Figure 8.19   *Fish*

RESOURCES

YOUNG PEOPLE

Dass, Baba Hari. *A Child's Garden of Yoga*. Santa Cruz, CA. Srirama Publishing. 1980.
Luby, Thai. *Children's Yoga with Animals*. Video, can be ordered from *Yoga Journal*.
Nelson-Burford, Annabelle . *How To Focus the Distractible Child*. Saratoga CA R&E Publishers. 1985.
Stewart, Mary and Kathy Phillips. *Yoga for Children*. New York, NY: Fireside. 1993.
_____ "Yoga for Kids", *Yoga Journal*. Sept./Oct. 1993. p/76-83

MENSTRUAL DISORDERS

Iyengar B.K.S. *Light On Yoga*. New York: Shocken Books, 1966.
Iyengar, Geeta S., *Yoga: A Gem for Women*: New Delhi: Allied, 1983.
McMullen, Jane. "Yoga and the Menstrual Cycle," *Yoga Journal*, Jan/Feb 1990. p 65-67, 91.

OLDER ADULTS

American Alliance of Health Physical Education, Recreation and Dance; Council on Aging and
        Adult Development. 1900 Association Drive, Reston, VA 22091.
"We're Having our Say..." *AARP Bulletin*. Feb/Mar. 1994. p. 20 & 12.
Birkel, Dee Ann and Susan Birkel Freitag. *Forever Fit: Step by Step Program of Physical Activity for Older Adults*.
        New York, Plenum Publishing, Insight Press. 1991.
Christensen, Alice and David Rankin. *Easy Does It Yoga : For Older People*. San Francisco CA
        Harper & Row Publishers. 1979.
Delany, Sarah and A. Elizabeth Delany with Amy Hill Hearth. *Having Our Say; The Delany Sisters; First 100 Years*.
        New York: Kodansha International. 1993.
_____ *The Delany Sisters' Book of Everyday Wisdom*. New York. Kodansha America, 1994.
Moore, Blake. "Yoga at 80". *Yoga Journal*, July/August 1995. p.26.
Stewart, Mary. *Yoga over Fifty*. New York, NY: Fireside. 1994.
Wakefield, Dan. "Be Old Now: Ram Dass." *Yoga Journal*. October, 1995. p. 66-73,138.
Ward, Susan Winter. VIDEO *Yoga for the Young at Heart: Gentle Stretching Exercises for Seniors*. Venice Ca.
        Healing Arts.

PREGNANCY

Arndt, Jennie. *Pre and Post Natal Yoga.* Video tape, 1-800-876-7798.

Balaskas, Janet. *Preparing for Birth with Yoga.* Rockport, MA: Element Books, Inc. 1994.

Goldstein, Leslie. *Relax with Yoga During Pregnancy,* Nityanada Institute. Audio tape with
foldout guide. 1-800-876-7798.

Jordan, Sandra. *Yoga for Pregnancy,* St. New York. Martins Press, 1987.

Lasater, Judith. *Relax and Renew.* Berkeley, CA. Rodmell Press, 1995.

_____"Yoga for Pregnancy," *Yoga Journal,* Jan/Feb. 1994, p. 88-98.

Moline, Peg. "Mama," *Fit Pregnancy,* Spring 1995, p. 52-59.

Music tapes for infants and children:
LULLABY FOR THE HEARTS OF SPACE, Kevin Braheny 42b-6 Pyramid Books and New-Age
Collection. 35 Congress St. P.O. Box 48 Salem, MA 01970.
LULLABY RIVER A04430   Red Rose Galleries, P.O. Box 1859, Burlingame, CA 94011
800-451-LOVE

VIDEO

St. Charles, Elize. *"Modern Moves for Pregnancy Fitness,"* Elize St. Charles & Associates, Los Gatos, CA 1990

VISUAL CONCERNS

Marantz-Henig, Robin and Judith Groch. "Too Close for Comfort." *American Health-Fitness of Body and Mind.*
April 1985, p. 62-71.

WHEELCHAIR

Brosnan, Barbara. *Yoga for Handicapped People.* London. Souvenir Press, 1982.

Bell, Lorna and Eudora Seyfer. *Gentle Yoga.* Cedar Rapids, Iowa. Igram Press, 1982.

Hall, Rosemary. "Seated Sun Salutation," *Yoga Journal ,* March/April, 1986.

Therapeutic Use of Yoga

> *We need to learn to know and appreciate our bodies as a collection of forces working together as one.*
> .... **Ilse Middendorf and Juerg A. Roffler**
> **"The Breathing Self" in**
> *The Journal of The International Association of Yoga Therapists Vol 5*

The time is NOW-hatha yoga is being recognized for what it has to offer in a variety of healing situations. One of the best kept "secrets " that persisted throughout the 70s and 80s was how the practice of yoga was helping people in yoga classes all over the world. The practice of yoga was waiting to be discovered and waiting for technology to develop the tools to measure its accomplishments in a variety of ways. This is happening now in the 90s. Those of us who have been teaching hatha yoga for thirty years or more knew that yoga was making a difference in people's lives. We also knew that the yoga books we used as references made these claims. The scientific proof is now forth coming. This unit will discuss these latest developments in yoga's long history.

Some examples of this acceptance are: as reported in the *Washington Post,* June 26, 1992, the National Institutes of Health received a $2 million congressional appropriation to establish the "Office for the Study of Unconventional Medical Practices." Their charge was to "more adequately explore and evaluate these unconventional medical practices." Many of the "alternative practices" here in the United States are ancient and honored traditions in other cultures, e.g. acupuncture, ayurvedic medicine, visualization, etc. The medical profession thus began a research program to better understand mind-body medicine.

As a result of the foresight of the astronaut, Edgar Mitchell, the organization entitled The Institute of Noetic Sciences, previously discussed in unit 6, was established in 1973 as a research foundation, educational institution and a membership organization. This organization funded some of the early research that documented the strong connection between the body, mind and innerself. They publish the quarterly

Noetic Sciences Review, and *Bulletin.* Their membership organization has over 30,000 members worldwide. Throughout the intervening years the field of "psychoneuroimmunology" continued to unfold and many people from a variety of backgrounds from physics to psychology and from medicine to sports became involved. In 1993, The Fetzer Institute, in Kalamazoo, MI, began publishing the quarterly networking resource for mind-body health study groups entitled *Mind-Body Health News.*

In 1994 the *Mental Medicine Update*: The Mind/Body Medicine Newsletter was published by The Center for Health Sciences, a branch of The Institute for the Study of Human Knowledge in Los Altos, CA. The major news magazines such as *U.S. News & World Report* have printed articles about wellness lifestyles that had their origins in yoga and related areas of mind/body therapies.

The pinnacle was reached when, in 1993, Bill Moyers hosted a 5 1/2 hour television series on public broadcasting entitled *Healing and the Mind*. The series was underwritten by the Fetzer Institute, with support from Mutual of America Life Insurance Company, Laurance S. Rockefeller, the John D. and Catherine T. Mac Arthur Foundation, and the Nathan Cummings Foundation. Educational materials were made available (free of charge) that included a sixteen page *Teacher's Resource Guide* written by the staff and associates of the Institute of Noetic Sciences and a twenty-four page illustrated *Viewer's Guide.* Videocassettes of the series were made available and the day after the second program aired all had been sold and there was a waiting list to order them. Doubleday published the book, *Healing And The Mind,* which was on the best seller list. This response indicated that our society was eager and more than ready to learn about "The Mystery of Chi," "The Mind Body Connection," "Healing From Within," "The Art of Healing," and "Wounded Healers," the titles of the programs. The entire series was aired again in 1994 and is usually available at libraries.

Many books have appeared in the area of self-help that encourage people to become an active participant in their healing process. Many of these books have been previously mentioned in this book or will be in this unit. Andrew Weil, M.D., has written *Spontaneous Healing,* in which he champions the body's intrinsic ability to heal from within"that should be the basis of medical practice." His book presents an eight-week program of modifying lifestyle to increase the healing power that includes healthy diet, exercise, even making time for flowers, music and art (USA Today, June 22, 1995 . 6D).

As you read further in this unit you will begin to respect the common thread which is at the base of the programs that incorporates yoga as a therapy. Basic to all is the approach that the person who has a condition is assisted in enpowering themself to be a major part of the healing process or in accepting their life at that moment. They are encouraged to trust their own self. By learning yoga, they are learning more about themselves, and by learning more they are gaining respect for their self, and in doing that they move to the next step of taking a more active role in their situation and how they are living their life. They are being offered the opportunity to listen to their own inner wisdom.

Yoga teachers, have also seen the need for a broader use of yoga as a therapy. Dr. Leroy Perry, the founder of the International Sportsmedicine Institute in west Los Angeles, established a yoga therapy department in 1985. Larry Payne serves as the director, Mara Carrico as associate director, a registered nurse, a clinical psychologist and experienced yoga teachers are members of their staff. They have worked with celebrities such as Wilt Chamberlain, Jane Fonda, Barbra Streisand, Jack Nicholson, and Warren Beatty. They focus on yoga therapy as a "work-in" not a "work-out" and emphasize it as a self-help program.

In 1990, a group of yoga teachers formed the International Association of Yoga Therapists, which publishes *The Journal of The International Association of Yoga Therapists.* Larry Payne, mentioned above, is the publisher and the board of directors is composed of the world's leading yoga teachers.

The organizations, authors, and yoga teachers will be mentioned later in this unit as we now begin to explore the relationship between yoga and the conditions that are listed. Refer to the resource section at the end of this unit for a listing of reference materials.

ADDICTIONS

A growing number of recovery activists are turning to the ancient discipline of yoga to bring the body into the 12 steps approach.
. . . D. Patrick Miller.
" The Case of the Missing Body,"
***Yoga Journal,* Jan/Feb 1995.**

There are many underlying causes for a person's tendency to become addicted to a substance that brings about instant gratification such as food, cigarettes, alcohol or illegal drugs. It is a complicated scene involving genes, dysfunctional family units, lifestyle pressures such as stress and economic settings as well as lack of knowledge about the harmful effects of a substance that can lead one to an addicted state. Many people have been helped with their addiction when yoga was introduced to them. It appears that a respect for the physical body is enhanced by doing the yoga asanas and pranayama. Thus a desire to take better care of the physical body develops. As a spin off, the benefits from relaxation, imagery and music then come into play. Often people with an addiction are not comfortable with focusing on the inner self and will attempt to deny their feelings by escaping with the addiction. By being led through the gentle coping mechanisms taught in yoga, such as using the breath to calm oneself, an addicted person can cope better with a daily trauma or a crisis.

An indication of the growing significance of the use of yoga as a treatment mode is illustrated by the clinical study of hatha yoga in substance abuse treatment being done at Harvard Medical School through the support of the National Institute of Health

In 1973 in Tucson, Arizona at the 3HO (Happy, Healthy and Holy Organization) a residential treatment program was developed. People coming here consisted of alcoholics, cigarette smokers, recreational drug users, people with weight problems, relationship difficulties and stress problems. At the center they did hatha yoga, mantra-chanting, and pranayama. They also had opportunities for counseling and massage and ate vegetarian meals to assist with detoxification and healing. People would stay from one week to one month (or longer if necessary). A survey of the graduates between 1983 to 1986 indicated a recovery rate of 91%. This center was designed for those who wanted to change and were willing to work to make it happen. This center closed in 1995 but there is still a need for this type of facility.

I was asked to teach an introductory hatha yoga class to young teenage girls who were sent by a court order to a addiction rehabilitation center. This was one of the most touching yoga sharing opportunities of my life. The young women absolutely enjoyed the 2 hour class and expressed their thanks with hugs and letters written to me. Their supervisors were amazed at their positive responses.

The pranayama practices bring to a smokers attention the state of their lungs. Gay Hendrick in his book, *Conscious Breathing,* chronicles one client who was instructed to do the deep breath, yoga complete breath - using the diaphragm, and the alternate nostril breath continuously under supervision "until her cheeks began to pinken, a sign to me that fresh energy was penetrating the cells. Smokers' skin takes on a yellow or gray cast as the result of oxygen deprivation; as soon as (she) broke through to a healthier skin tone, I took her over to the mirror and showed her". I asked her to do the 'three Foundation lessons' three times each day, not stopping until she saw pink in her cheeks" (p. 133). Also, when she got a craving for a cigarette, she was to do the alternate nostril breath until the craving went away.

There are no specific precautions and recommendations for those with addictions in regards to their hatha yoga practice. The use of affirmations is a positive way of reenforcing positive attitudes. The book *Stretch & Surrender,* by Annalisa Cunningham, who is a person in recovery, is written as a guide to yoga, health and relaxation for other people in recovery. She incorporates a fitting affirmation with a yoga pose - as an example: for the **Triangle** - " I am filled with acceptance and love."

At the Bay Cove Human Services, in Boston MA, a methadone maintenance detox treatment center, some of the addicts-turned yogis "felt that the practice of yoga facilitated a release of physical and emotional tension that was more direct and immediate than ordinary psychotherapy" as reported by Tom

LaSalvia, director of the study (*Yoga Journal.* Jan/Feb 1995 p. 72). In summarizing, hatha yoga has much to offer to those overcoming an addiction. All of the poses would be fine to do, with emphasis on the breath, imagery and relaxation.

ARTHRITIS

Hatha yoga poses are recommended for those with arthritis. The manner in which the asanas are done is very helpful to those with arthritis. The Arthritis Foundation and many physicians recognize that exercise helps to improve the condition. Patients are encouraged to participate in exercises that increase muscle strength as that can help protect the joints. Even the cardiovascular exercises such as walking, swimming, water exercises and low/non impact aerobic dance are now being recommended for those who can enjoy it. James Fries M.D., associate director of Stanford Arthritis Center, says that "body systems including the joints, work better when they are used then when they are not used" (*Physician and Sports Medicine,* Jan. 1990, p.123). In the resource section there is a listing of arthritis programs, articles and the address of the Arthritis Foundation where you can obtain more information.

Precautions:

1. Don't do weight bearing asanas that jar the joints.

Recommendations:

1. Do the poses in a slow, controlled static stretch.
2. Move through the fullest range of motion of which the joint is capable .
3. Use the breath to help with the flow of energy and to increase circulation.
4. Visualize the affected area moving easily with no pain or discomfort to assist the body to become stronger and healthier.
5. Visualize your body in a perfect skeletal alignment with strong, flexible muscles holding your skeleton together in its perfect alignment.
6. Try doing the standing yoga poses in a pool (water at 83 to 88 degrees F).
7. If you have rheumatoid arthritis, wait until later in the day to practice as the morning stiffness will have abated.
8. If you have osteoarthritis, practice earlier in the day before the wear and tear of the days activities have tired the affected joints.

9. If you are experiencing pain 2 hours after your yoga session then you need to scale down or modify your exercises.
10. It is very important to do the preparation poses you enjoy to warm up and also cool down.
11. Use the necktie to assist you in moving into the yoga asanas
12. Light massage and heat or ice can help with pain, as well as acupuncture

Recommended Asanas for Arthritis

Preparation Poses: For Warm Up and Cool Down
All poses presented in Unit 3 are suitable but if there is an area of your body that is bothered by them do the pose very gently. If there is pain, DON'T do the pose.

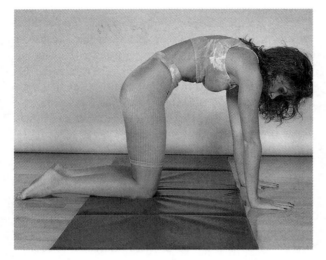

Figure 9.1   *Cat*

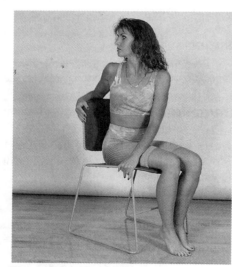

Figure 9.2   *Spinal Twist*

ASANAS
1. Mountain Pose (Fig. 3.13)
2. Cobra: Modification - if palms can not go flat to the mat make fists instead (Fig. 3.14)
3. Cat: Same modification as above (Fig. 9.1)
4. Dog: Same modification as above (Fig. 3.23)
5. Head of the Cow: Use necktie if needed. This pose is in the Arthritis Foundation Videotape of their PACE program (People With Arthritis Can Exercise) (Fig. 3.19)
6. Shoulderstand: Whichever variation feels good (Fig. 3.25)
7. Spinal Twist in chair (Fig. 9.2)
8. Crocodile Routine (Unit 6) of Swami Dev Murti, as it is wonderful for the spine and the laughter part is helpful with pain control
9. Almost all of the asanas are suitable if YOU feel comfortable doing them.Some may be more difficult to do than others such as the following: Lunge, Plank, Spinal Twist, Full Locust

ASTHMA

> *The emotional and physical states*
> *can be altered*
> *by changing the breathing pattern*
>
> **. . . Wilheim Reich (German psychologist)**

Gay Hendricks, Ph.D., the author of *Conscious Breathing,* tells of his work with asthmatics since the 1970s. He has helped hundreds to retrain themselves to breathe correctly and thus helps them to handle the emotions that can trigger an asthma attack. He is a counseling psychologist and teaches his clients the abdominal breath, the alternate nostril breath and how to lengthen and deepen the exhalation by allowing a candle flame to flicker but not be extinguished on the exhalation. He also teaches an activity that coordinates the breath with a body movement by making a figure eight arm movement in front of the body with the eyes focusing on the hands. This movement is to be done with awareness of your movement **and** your breath and where you may feel "stuck." These practices allow the asthmatic to gain some control of their breath and to do activities that are beneficial for their lungs.

A medical doctor, P. K. Vedanthan, conducted a 12-week study of patients with mild asthma. He found that practicing yoga three times a week resulted in a significantly higher degree of relaxation, better exercise tolerance, less panic associated with asthma symptoms, a more positive attitude, less exercise-induced lung spasms, better lung function and decreased use of medication especially adrenergic inhalers. The asthmatics were taught a combination of pranayama and relaxation techniques. The yoga shoulder stand was especially associated with better breathing as the chest is opened and the diaphragm is strengthened. Dr. Vedanthan, an allergist in Fort Collins, CO, emphasizes that by calming the mind and relaxing the body you are reducing the stress level and therefore may also be reducing the physical symptoms as well.

The results of another research study with asthma suffers was reported in *The Lancet* (vol. 335, no. 8702). This study conducted by Virendra Singh, M.D., found that the use of pranayama exercises in those with mild asthma led to overall improvement in lung function equal to or greater than that obtained through hypnosis or the use of low-dose inhaled cortocosteroids. It is thought that the yoga exercises helped increase the bronchial dilation and the lung's efficiency.

BACK PROBLEMS

> *Everyone that walks through my door*
> *is a candidate for yoga.*
> *Yoga helps every single type of injury*
> *or problem expecially neck and back pain.*
>
> **. . . Lisa Ann McCall.**
> **Dallas physical therapist in**
> **"A Yen for Yoga"**
> *USAir Magazine* **March 1992**

Back ache and pain is probably the single most expensive problem that affects adults. It is estimated that four out of five Americans have back problems - approximately 200 million at some time in their life will be bothered. Each year roughly another 5 million will strain or sprain their back. It is estimated that 83% of the problems are caused by muscular weakness, tension and stress. The lack of flexibility of the back from the head to the toes, weak abdominal muscles, bad posture habits and lack of proper lifting and carrying techniques are also prevalent causes. This is where yoga comes in. Overall posture is stressed whether in a sitting, standing or lying position. Yoga asanas are well known for improving the flexibility of the body. The relaxation portion of a yoga class also has beneficial effect on those with back problems.

In yoga the spine is very important. To help maintain strength and flexibility the back needs to be moved gently in all six directions daily - bending forward, gently arching the back, leaning to the right and the left and gently twisting to the right and the left. The routine presented will accomplish this.

Fortunately for those who are bothered by back problems there is a book written by a medical doctor and senior Iyengar Yoga teacher. Mary Pullig Schatz, M.D., has written *Back Care Basics* which is a source of information on how the back is designed to function in a normal manner and how to determine what is going on when a problem is present. She also explains with diagrams, photos of yoga poses, and adaptations of poses what people can do to help themselves.

The *Men's Health,* October, 1991 issue, printed the results of a survey of 492 back-pain sufferers in which YOGA INSTRUCTORS were listed as "number 1" for providing " Moderate to Dramatic Long-Term Relief." 96% of those responding to the survey placed them first. Even when yoga is not

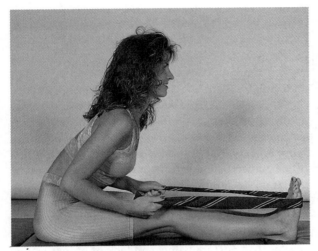

Figure 9.3   *Sitting Forward Bend*

presented strictly as a therapy mode for back problems, people notice that their backs have become more flexible, the muscles stronger, and posture is improved.

Precautions:

1. The **Full Locust** can aggravate an existing problem in the lumbar area. Do with caution after back has become stronger. Don't lift legs very high.
2. Do not do **Standing Forward Bend** if there is discomfort in the lumbar area or have a problem with the sciatic nerve. It is better to do the **Sitting Forward Bend** (Fig. 9.3).

Recommendations:

1. Notice how your back feels as you do the poses. Notice if one side is tighter than the other.
2. Do the routine for backs daily.
3. Do some of the preparation poses at the beginning and end of the day.
4. Vary your sleeping posture and don't use a large pillow as it pushes the head forward When lying on your side support the bent top leg with a pillow.
5. Observe your postural habits when carrying, sit ting and standing.

Recommended Asanas for Backs:

1. Moon Salute (Fig. 3.35)
2. Body rolls (Fig. 3.3)
3. Alternate Leg stretch (Fig. 3.12)
4. Pelvic Tilt
5. Feldenkrais knee overs (Fig. 3.10)
6. Cobra (Fig. 3.14AB)
7. 1/2 Locust (Fig. 3.15)
8. Fetus (Fig. 3.16) or Knee to chest (Fig. 3.17)
9. Yoga Sit Back and Up (Fig. 3.24)
10. Abdominal Lift (Fig. 3.31)

The Crocodile Routine in Unit 6 is most beneficial as the back muscles are freed from some of the effects of gravity. Doing the gentle exercises horizontally means that no vertebrae or muscle is holding up another, and thus the back is allowed to twist more easily.

SCOLIOSIS

This is a condition in the spine which allows the vertebrae to curve to the side, also affects the rib cage, shoulders and hips, thus changing the center of gravity. Adolescence is a time during which structural scoliosis, which is an unequal growth of the two sides of the vertebrae, develops. Functional scoliosis develops usually from poor posture habits and unbalanced activity, such as always carrying your book bag or back pack on the same shoulder. Yoga exercises can help with functional scoliosis and with structural scoliosis if it is identified soon enough.

Precautions:

The **Headstand** should be done with care and supervised by an experienced yoga teacher.

Recommendations:

1. Take the pressure off the concave side of the spine (Fig.9.4).
2. Flex the spine in the opposite direction of the concave curve.
3. Twisting the spine can also help relieve the stretch and tension on the convex side.
4. Always visualize <u>extending and lengthening</u> the spine.
5. Hang from the knees on a bar or a jungle gym to allow the back to stretch and relieve the compression between the vertebrae.
6. Practice pranayama to help keep the thoracic area flexible.
7. See the resource section for articles in the *Yoga Journal* for those with scoliosis.

Recommended Asanas for Scoliosis:

1. Cat (Fig. 3.21)
2. Shoulder & Back Stretch at Wall or Barre (Fig. 3.7)
3. Fetus (Fig. 9.5)
4. Downward Facing Dog (Fig. 3.23)
5. Triangle: do first on the concave side, repeat to the convex side and a third time on the concave side (Fig. 3.29).
6. Spinal Twist in chair (Fig. 9.2)
7. Triangle Twist: do on concave side as it will then derotate the spine (Fig. 3.30)
8. Locust: strengthens the erector spinae of the back and the hamstrings in the legs. (Fig. 4.4)
9. Shoulderstand (Fig. 3.25)
10. Relaxation pose with a conscious effort to line the spine as straight as possible (Fig.6.1)

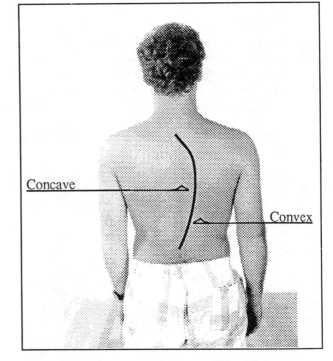

Figure 9.4   *Concave and Convex Side of Spine*

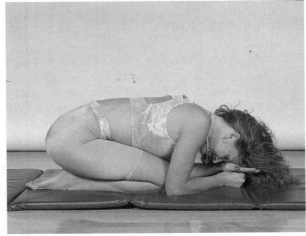

Figure 9.5   *Fetus*

NECK INJURY

Many people have injured their neck in a variety of ways. A common injury is "whiplash" which can leave the muscles of the neck sore and weakened. The alignment of the cervical vertebrae is not always corrected and can lead to tension and muscle fatigue. Yoga poses can assist in strengthening these muscles. You should have permission from your physician to begin exercising. You may have been given a set of exercises to do, and if so, share them with your yoga teacher.

Precautions:

1. Do not do any poses which will hyperflex the neck such as the **Shoulderstand** on a flat surface
2. When doing the **Fish**, you lift your 12-15 pound head, and you may be overloading the neck muscles- DON'T lift the head if it causes pain but simply lower the head tucking the chin to the chest (Fig. 9.6)
3. DON'T do the **Headstand Hang** or the **Headstand** without careful supervision.

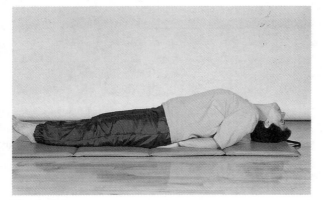

Figure 9.6

Recommendations:

1. Always be aware of how you are holding your head over your spine. If you get in the habit of monitoring the head and have it centered over the strong bones of the spine there is a lot less work for the neck muscles to do
2. Do gentle stretches and turns frequently during the day
3. Don't sleep on a large pillow as that pushes your head forward. You can purchase a pillow that is designed to fit the natural curve of the cervical spine
4. Trade neck massages with friends

5. When studying, typing, drawing etc., take frequent breaks to change position and do some of the stretches recommended in the following routine.
6. Keep the head in a straight alignment at all times- for example keep the chin and not the cheek on the mat when doing the **1/2 Locust**

Recommended Asanas for Necks:

1. Neck stretches (Fig. 3.1) and neck turns (Fig. 3.2)
2. Chest Expansion (Fig. 3.20)
3. Head lift and turn: strengthens the front of the neck. (Fig. 3.9)
4. Fish (Fig. 3.26)
5. Dog (Fig. 3.23)
6. Dolphin: maintain most of the weight with the arms and gradually shift some to the neck, being very aware of how the neck feels when you do that. Stop if it hurts. (Fig. 3.34)

CANCER

The purpose of life is to grow in wisdom and to learn to love better. If life serves these purposes, then health serves these purposes and illness serves them as well, because illness is part of life.
. . . Rachel Naomi Remen M.D.
& Medical Director at the *Commonweal* - about cancer patients, *Noetic Sciences Collection*

Cancer can be thought of as a disease process at the cellular level- it is not simply ONE disease. It can be thought of as a group of about 100 diseases that can affect any organ of the body. So, consequently, the question is raised, what can be done to keep the cellular level in a healthy state so that the cell development and growth will not become abnormal? There is no simple answer. All cells need oxygen - the lungs need to be healthy so that the carbon dioxide-oxygen exchange can take place in all areas of the lungs. A low fat diet is recommended as research has found that cancer cells and tumors thrive on fat. Viruses, free radicals, chemicals and radiation can upset the normal cell. The body's systems of resistance need to be strengthened. We need to take into consideration how strong the immune system is; the nutritional intake and absorption efficiency; and how stress affects the hormone level, the central nervous system and the autonomic nervous system. There is a theory that helps explain the "host resistance" to disease -the psychoneuroimmunology (PNI) paradigm. Research has shown that there is a constant communication between the immune system and the brain about cancer cells. The immune system and nervous system interaction seems to be controlled by the mind.

Yoga can play a beneficial role by offering the stress reduction practices of relaxation, meditation, and visualization. The practice of pranayama can enhance the basic health of the cells through an adequate supply of oxygen. Exercise is recommended as a coping activity - and yoga can be done with a gentle approach so that those undergoing Western medical treatments of chemotherapy and radiation can practice. When any person is beginning yoga they are committing themselvs to a practice that will potentially result in something positive for their entire state of health. Those with cancer are no different. As mentioned in Unit 6, Stress, it is how you perceive an event that affects your stress response to that event.

In the small town of Bolinas, CA, at the *Commonweal,* the "Cancer Help Program" was established in 1985. This is a residential program offered eight times a year for eight participants a session. Michael Lerner, the founder, says "The goal of the Commonweal Cancer Help Program is to help people navigate the life passage called cancer." The participants have a week-long immersion in health education, vegetarian diet, massage, stress reduction, exercise, deep relaxation, creative imagery and yoga asana practice in the style of Swami Satchidananda, all of this with ocean air, healing silence, a caring environment and group support (Yoga Journal, Sept, / Oct. 1990, p. 64). The Commonweal also was featured on the PBS *Healing and the Mind's,* episode the "Wounded Healers."

People who are diagnosed with cancer now have a much larger support system to tap into. No one needs to feel they are in this "alone." As an example, there is a nonprofit organization, "The Cancer Support Community" that offers a range of services and support to hundreds of cancer patients a week. For information see resources.

HEART DISEASE

> *Two things are bad for the heart-*
> *running uphill and running down people.*
> . . . **Bernard Gimbel**

Dean Ornish, M.D., and colleagues conducted landmark studies in the effort to reverse heart disease, using hatha yoga, diet and stress reduction. Their results have received considerable coverage in the press and on television. This program had its origins back in 1984 when Ornish and Dr. Sandra McLanahan collaborated on a trial project using yoga exercises and a low-fat, low-cholesterol diet with twenty-three Baylor College of Medicine heart patients. Their findings showed that each patient's heart had become a more efficient pump, and with the yoga and dietary changes their tension had lessened. The promising results of this early study led to another one which resulted in his first book, *Stress , Diet and Your Heart,* published in 1986. Dr Ornish received his medical training at Harvard and Baylor College of Medicine and is the head of the Preventive Medicine Research Institute in Sausalito, CA, and is a faculty member of the University of California at San Francisco. He is also one of the advisors to the National Institute of Health Office of the Study of Unconventional Medical Practices. I have been following closely Dr. Ornish and his program since I first read about it in the *Yoga Journal* September/October issue of 1989 and again in the March/April issue of 1991. With the publication of his research project and findings in the July 21, 1990 medical publication *The Lancet,* his program of reversing coronary heart disease finally was recognized more broadly by the medical community.

Dr. Ornish presented his research findings at Ball State University in September 1992 as a part of a week long "Universe City" series of enrichment activites and lectures for our university community. The nation's largest provider of health care insurance for individuals, Mutual of Omaha, announced in 1993 that it would reimburse patients who take part in the "Dr. Ornish Reversal Program." They estimate that the cost is one tenth the price of conventional coronary care. In 1995 hospitals in- Omaha, NE.; Des Moines, IA; New York,NY; Columbia, S.C.; and Ft. Lauderdale, Fl, began offering the program to patients. The teams of cardiologists, dieticians, exercise physiologists, nurses, psychologists, stress management instructors and yoga teachers are trained at the nonprofit Preventive Medicine Research Center. Ornish's goal with this project is to save lives and as a result also save dollars.

The "Program for Reversing Heart Disease" consists of the following:

> **The Reversal Diet** which allows only 10% of the total calories to come from fat, 5 milligrams of cholesterol per day, no high saturated fat foods (such as nuts, seeds, avocados), no oils, no animal products except egg whites, nonfat yogurt and nonfat milk, and no caffeine, MSG or stimulants.
>
> **The Stress Reduction and Increased Intimacy** approach utilizes yoga asanas and pranayama, progressive relaxation, guided visualization, meditation, training in communication, and opportunities for compassion, group support and sharing.
>
> **The Moderate Exercise Program** requires the participants to walk 30 minutes a day or 1 hour three times a week; to learn to exercise safely; and to chose a type of exercise you enjoy.
>
> **The Program to Stop Addictive Behaviors** targets overuse of alcohol or tobacco, and being a workaholic. They are encouraged to seek out the underlying cause of the addiction and work toward developing healthy behaviors.

The hatha yoga portion of the program is described in his book *Dr. Dean Ornish's Program for Reversing Heart Disease,* chapter 7, "Opening your Heart to Your Feelings and to Inner Peace." The participants are taught 13 of the basic poses and the Sun Salute, followed by deep relaxation. The pranayama they are taught consists of the abdominal breath, the complete deep breath, bellows breath and the alternate nostril breath. As mentioned above they are also instructed in visualization.

Dr. Ornish's first two books have large sections of delicious, low-fat, low-cholesterol vegetarian recipes. His third book, *Eat More, Weigh Less,* came about because in his research studies the patients lost an average of twenty-two pounds even though they were eating more food, more frequently than before they entered the studies. So, the Life Choice diet evolved, which is rich in vitamins, and very low in oxidants that can harm the DNA. The recipes in his books have been collected from friends and chefs. Some recipes are traditional favorites that have been adapted to meet his low-fat, no animal product, low-cholesterol, high nutrient requirements.

Dr. Ornish and his belief in an alternative way to treat heart disease that approached the problem at the causal level rather than at the symptomatic level is an inspiration to all. His approach is now being taught and his ideas have helped others broaden their way of

thinking. The International Association of Yoga Therapists sponsored a *Yoga with Heart* workshop in October 1995 with Ornish's colleagues, Larry Schweritz, as guest speaker and Amy Kline-Gage, Judith Lasater, and Nischala Joy Devi as workshop leaders. Dr. Ornish has spent over seventeen years of his career as a cardiologist seeking a program that worked. For those readers who are interested in his program check the resource section at the end of this chapter and watch the *Healing and the Mind,* PBS television program entitled " The Mind Body Connection."

An emphasis should be placed on using the breath to improve the health of the heart. Gay Hendricks, in his book, *Conscious Breathing,* reports on research done in The Netherlands with heart attack patients. One group was taught to do diaphragmatic breathing while the second group had no breathing training. The groups were followed for two years with the result that the first group had no more heart attacks while seven of the twelve patients in the second group had a second heart attack. The recommendation from the Dutch study is that people should be taught to shift from chest and/or mouth breathing to abdominal breathing as it may nourish the body with more oxygen so the heart is not having to work as hard to move less-oxygenated blood through the body (*Conscious Breathing* p 16-17).

PAIN

> *Go from just existing - to LIVING.*
> . . . **Jon Kabat-Zinn, M.D.** in
> *Healing and the Mind* PBS television program

What is PAIN? Pain is a warning signal for the body that something is not right and needs attention. Finding the cause of the pain is the first step and then you can deal with it through treatment . When pain becomes chronic and can not be alleviated, it can tire the body and cause stress. What can be done? Well, one man had an idea and he proceeded to develop the idea and see if it would bring about positive results. Jon Kabat-Zinn M.D. (who has been a long time practitioner of yoga and meditation) established a Yoga-based Stress Reduction Clinic in 1979-80 at the University of Massachusetts Medical Center in Worcester. "I found hatha yoga to be one of the great gifts to humanity. There is no better way to understand the workings of the body. That, along with Buddhist meditative practice, is the absolute core that informs every aspect of our work in the Stress Reduction Clinic.

Hatha isn't about turning your body into an elaborate pretzel; it's about living your life in balance between *ha* and *tha,* between self and totality, so that everything in life is a manifestation of yoga" (*Yoga Journal,* March/April 1995, p.67).

The people Kabat-Zinn began working with were the ones who had tried all other avenues of medical treatment and still were in pain. The program consists of eight consecutive weeks of two and a half hour yoga/breathing/ relaxation classes plus forty-five minutes of at home meditation practice daily. They also are required to attend a seven-hour silent retreat during the sixth week. The participants are given audio tapes for their at home meditation/relaxation time. After they have completed the program, the participants have a one-hour individual follow-up interview. Throughout the program they are encouraged to be self-motivated and to use a gentle non-competitive approach. One of the participants was interviewed along with Kabat-Zinn on "Oprah" and had this to say- "This is probaby a little confusing, but I focus right on the pain so that I can accept it. I have to look right at it so that I can get to the other side." In the research findings about the participants that have been published in the *Clinical Journal of Pain,* the *American Journal of Psychiatry* and the *Journal of Behavioral Medicine* 90% interviewed for the program enroll, 85% of those who start also finish, and 91% are maintaining their at-home practice at the three-month follow-up. Were they helped? Yes, as the results show of those who were suffering from chronic pain for an average of six to seven years: 30 to 55%- greatly improved, and 60-72% moderate or great improvement.

The program at Worcester, MA, also was featured on *The Healing and the Brain,* PBS television program entitled "Healing from Within". Dr. Kabat-Zinn, is the author of two books: *Full Catastrophe Living: Using the Wisdom of Your Body and Mind to Face Stress, Pain and Illness* (Delta, 1990), and *Wherever You Go, There You Are: Mindfulness Meditation in Everyday Life* (Hyperion, 1994). Dr. Kabat-Zinn has always been straightforward with the fact that the program consists of Eastern disciplines and never attempted to camoflage them as anything else. As a result of the success of this project, Dr. Kabat-Zinn has consulted with other hospitals in establishing Stress/Pain Reduction Clinics. Most of the large cities in the United States now have a hospital - based clinic of this type.

Many hospitals also have a "Laughter Cart" or team that provides joke books, videos, and cassettes tapes to the patients. As mentioned earlier in Unit 6, Norman Cousins was the first to share the benefits of laughter in healing and pain control with the world. Since 1979 this concept is now widely accepted in the medical community. At nursing conferences, there are sessions on "How to be a Clown," and other laughter producing tactics that can be used in a hospital setting. Bernie Siegell, M.D,. who was another pioneer in the mind/body healing connection has an audiotape on "Humor and Healing" (see resources).

RESOURCES

Therapeutic Approaches

Achterberg, Jeanne Ph.D, Barbara Dossey, Leslie Kolkmeier. *Rituals of Healing; Using Imagery for Health and Wellness.* Bantam Books, New York. 1994.

Advances: The Journal of Mind-Body Health. The Fetzer Institute. 9292 West KL Avenue. Kalamazoo MI 49009.

Butera, Robert Jr. "A Vision of Yoga Therapy as Lifestyle Education," *The Journal of The International Association of Yoga Therapists.* vol 5. p. 42-45.

Chopra, Deepak, M.D. *Quantum Healing: Toward Perfect Health.* New York, NY Bantam. 1990.

_____*Perfect Health: The Complete Mind/Body Guide.* New York, NY. Harmony Books. 1991.

The Journal of the International Association of Yoga Therapists. 366 Edgewood Avenue, Mill Valley CA 94941, 415-381-982. Fax 415-381-5982.

Dacher, Elliott S. *PNI: The New Mind/Body Healing Program.* New York, NY Shoot Star. 1994.

Goleman Daniel and Joel Gurin. *Mind/Body Medicine: How to Use Your Mind for Better Health.* Consumer Reports Books, Yonkers, N.Y.: 1993.

Goodheart, Annette. Ph.D *Laugh Your Way to Health .* Videocassette.

Grossmann, John. "Your Emotions Can Help You fight Cancer, Heart Disease and More," *New Choices.* Feb. 1995. p. 24-27.

Hendricks, Gay, Ph.D. *Conscious Breathing.* Bantam Books, New York, 1995

Integrative Yoga Therapy for Body, Mind and Spirit, 305 Vista De Valle, Mill Valley, CA 94941.

Klein, Allen. *The Healing Power of Humor.* Los Angeles, CA.   J. P.Tarcher. 1989.

Lad, Vasant M.D. *Ayurveda: The Science of Life* . Six audio cassettes with booklet. Sounds True Catalog, 735 Walnut
    St. Dept SC8, Boulder, CO. 1-800-333-9185

Lee, Michael M.A. "The Call of Spirit: A Case Study in Phoenix Rising Yoga Therapy," *The Journal of the International
    Association of Yoga Therapists.*   Vol. 5. p. 34-36.1995.

Pelletier, Kenneth R. PhD. *Sound Mind, Sound Body: A New Model for Lifelong Health.*   New York, NY: Simon &
    Schuster. 1994

Woldenberg, Susan. "Yoga Therapy", *Yoga Journal.* Mar/Apr 1985, p. 46-49, & 51.

Addictions

Cunningham, Annalisa. *Stretch & Surrender.* Cambridge, Massachusetts, Rudra Press. 1992.

Lefton, Judith. "Yoga Therapy for Addictions," *Yoga Journal.* March/April 1990, p.25-30.

Miller, D. Patrick. "The Case of the Missing Body". *Yoga Journal.* Janurary/February 1995. p. 72-77.

Shepherd, Bliss. "Dealing with Our Addictions," *Yoga Journal.* November/December 1988, p. 49, 103.

Arthritis

Gach, Michael Reed. "Morning Stretches for Aching Joints," *Yoga Journal,* September/October 1989. P. 19-28.

Haslock, I. et al. "Measuring the effects of yoga in rheumatoid arthritis," *British Journal of Rheumatology.* August, 1994.
    vol 33. p. 787-8.

Samples, Pat. "Exercise Encouraged for People With Arthritis," . *Physician and Sports Medicine.* Vol 18, No. 1 Janurary
    l990. p.123-125, 127.

Arthritis Foundation, Box 19000, Atlanta, GA 30326.

Fries, James M.D., and Kate Lorig. *The Arthritis Helpbook.* Stanford CA: Arthritis Center.

Asthma

"Better Breathing," *Prevention.* Vol. 43. Janurary 1991. P. 8-9.

Hendricks, Gay. Ph. D. *Conscious Breathing.* New York, NY: Bantam Books, 1995

Ingall, M. "Yoga Breathing Eases Asthma," *McCalls.* Vol. 118. March, 1991. p. 40.

Middendorf, Illse and Juerg A. Roffler. "The Breathing Self: The Experience of Breath as an Art to Healing Yourself."
The Journal of The International Association of Yoga Therapists. Vol. 5. 1995 p.13-18.

Middendorf, Illse. *The Perceptible Breath* (includes audio tapes). Berkeley CA. Somatic Resources. 1990.

Back Problems

Gunnell, Ellise. "A Yen For Yoga," *USAir Magazine.* March 1992 p. 86, 88-90.

Hatlett, Larry. "Hatha Yoga and Scoliosis," Y*oga Journal.* September/October 1982. p. 53-54.

Miller, Elise Browning. "Yoga for Scoliosis," *Yoga Journal.* May/June 1990. p. 66-75, 105-6.

Schatz, Mary Pullig, M.D. "Living With Your Lower Back," *Yoga Journal.* July/August 1984.

_____ *Back Care Basics.* , Berkeley CA. Rodmell Press,1992.

_____ "Back Care Basics: A Doctor's Gentle Yoga Program for Back and Neck Pain Relief," *The Journal of the
    International Association of Yoga Therapists.* vol 5. 1995.

Setterberg, Fred. "How I Got My Back Up," *In Health.* March/April 1990. p. 40-49.

Cancer

Cancer Smart.   Newsletter from Memorial Sloan-Kettering Cancer Center. PO Box 808, Yorktown Heights NY 10598-
    9932.

The Cancer Support Community, 401 Laurel Street. San Francisco, CA 94118. 415-929-7400.

Coping: Living with Cancer. Magazine, 219 North Carothers, Nashville, TN 37064.

Lerner, Michael. *Choice in Cancer.* Videotape. Commonweal, Box 316, Bolinas, CA 94924.

Le Shan, Lawrence. *Cancer as a Turning Point.* New York, NY. E. P. Dutton . 1994

Remen, Rachel N. and Michael Lerner. *Conversations at the Edge: The Art of Choice.* Videotape. Commonweal, Box 316,
    Bolinas, CA 94924.

Simonton, O.Carl M.D., and Reid Henson. *The Healing Journey; The Simonton Center Program for Achieving Physical,
    Mental, and Spiritual Health.* New York, NY. Bantam. 1994

Heart Disease

Andrews, Valerie. "Yoga and Your Heart," *Esquire*. Janurary. 1984, p. 116.

Lasater, Judith. "Yoga and Your Heart," *Yoga Journal*. September/Octtober. 1989, p. 13-15.

Ornish, Dean MD., et al. "The Lifestyle Heart Trial," *The Lancet*, :1990; Vol 336, p. 129-33.

_____ "Dr. Dean Ornish's Guide to A Healthy Heart," *Yoga Journal* . March/April 1991, p.50-53, 106-107.

_____ "Eat More, Weigh Less." *Yoga Journal*. November/December. 1993. p. 23-24, 27-28, &30.

_____ *Eat More, Weigh Less,* New York. Harper Collin Publishers, 1993

_____ *Dr. Dean Ornish's Program for Reversing Heart Disease.* Random House. New York,1990

_____ *Stress, Diet and Your Heart.* New York, NY: New American Library. 1986

Pain

Caudill, Margaret A MD, PhD. *Managing Pain Before It Manages You.* New York. NY. Guildford Pr. 1994.

Garfinkel, Perry. " Meditation Goes Mainstream," *Yoga Journal*. Issue 121, April 1995.

Kabat-Zinn, Jon M.D. *Full Catastrophe Living: Using the Wisdom of Your Body and Mind to Face Stress, Pain and Illness.* New York, NY: Delacorte Press. 1990.

_____ *Wherever You Go, There You Are: Mindfulness Meditation in Everyday Life.* New York, NY: Hyperion, 1994.

Ornstein, Robert Ph.D. and David S. Sobel, MD. "Managing Chronic Pain," *Mental Medicine Update; the Mind/Body Medicine Newsletter.* Vol IV, No 1, 1995.

Siegel, Bernie, M.D. "Humor and Healing." 90 minute videotape. Sounds True Catalog 735 Walnut St., Dept SC8, Boulder, C0 80302. 1-800-333-9185.

Yoga : Sports and Dance

> *Every athletic career, no matter how modest or lofty, is a journey.*
> *On any journey, we need a clear map, a sound vehicle and sufficient quality of fuel.*
> *The mind is the map, the body the vehicle and the emotions the fuel.*
>   . . . Dan Millman, *The Warrior Athlete.xiii*

Many champion athletes have enjoyed and benefitted from doing yoga - Jean Claude Killey, the French Olympic ski champion; the golfers Jack Nicklaus and Gary Player; boxer Sugar Ray Robinson; basketball player Kareem Abdul Jabbar; tennis player John McEnroe; and dancers Ruth St. Denis, Marge Champion, Shirley MacLaine and numerous others. Football teams such as the Washington Redskins and the Pittsburgh Steelers began doing yoga like stretches to prevent injuries. The reason they value yoga is that they see the benefits and positive effects in their athletic performance.

MUSCULAR/BREATHING BENEFITS

All atheletes notice improvement in their flexibility and their range of motion when they do hatha yoga. A greater awareness of their overall postural alignment will aid an athlete with the concentration needed for the correct postural alignment for their specific sport skills. All of the cells of the body need oxygen to adequately perform. Learning more efficent use of the breath will help with the energy/ oxygen level. Also, the calming breath such as the alternate nostril breath, will aid an athlete in being prepared for intense competition.

RELAXATION BENEFITS

The practice of relaxation in SHAVASANA, the corpse position, will carry over to a relaxed execution of a particular sports skill. A relaxed muscle moves more freely and easily. Being too tense can inhibit the flow of your movement. Bud Winter, the track coach at San Jose State from 1940-1970, brought attention to the value of relaxation in sports. His track athletes earned thirty-seven world records. At one time his runners held all ten world records for sprinting and made an outstanding showing for the United States at the 1968 Olympics in Mexico City. He had taken the relaxation techniques that he had helped develop at the United States Naval Aviation School at the Del Monte Pre-Flight center during World War II and applied them to coaching his track athletes. In the early research with the Navy pilots, they "found that in all sports and highly specialized skills, such as flying a plane, the greatest enemy to peak performance was hypertension- that is too much tension" (Winter, *Relax and Win,* p.4). They also discovered that one should relax the muscles that are not necessary to perform the task at hand. So Winter coached his atheletes to put out nine-tenths effort, as going all out at 100% caused "tying up," wasting their energy and causing the muscles to perform less efficiently. His athletes were determined mentally but stayed loose and relaxed physically. In his book, *Relax and Win,* he applies his technique to boxing, baseball, skiing, swimming, basketball, bowling, golf, tennis, soccer, football and track and field. Being relaxed also can speed up the reaction time, which is a key element in executing many sports skills.

MENTAL BENEFITS

The mind's involvement in sports performance has been gaining more attention. "Mental practice" is a form of imagery or visualization as discussed in unit 6. Video tapes have been made of the worlds best performers who executes athletic skills flawlessly. Then you view the tape and image yourself doing the identical movements. When you combine this "image" with being in a relaxed state you can enhance your performance. A *US News &World Report* article entitled "Mind & Body; The new science of performing at your peak," highlighted the growing awareness of the mental edge that comes when the brain is being utilized in performance (August, 1992). The article discusses the importance of the minds involvement in "psyching up," motivation, concentration, mental imagery and stress control. All of these important components can be enhanced through the practice of hatha yoga and pranayama.

This development of the tools of imagery and visualization doesn't have to end when an athletic career is over. Marilyn King, a member of two Olympic teams as a pentathlete, is the director of an organization *Beyond Sports*. Her goal for this organization is to aid people in extending the application of visualization to their daily life, and thus moving visualization into the broader arena of individual and social issues. King hopes to give young children the hope to imagine that they too could be a Mary Lou Retton and to help them " realize what desire, vision and commitment can accomplish" (*Noetic Sciences Collection.* p 340).

Bud Winter advises having a "mental set" such as being "cool and confident." This can help you with your sport performance. The following are examples of situations and "Mental Set" slogans from Bud Winters book.

Bud Winter's Mental Sets

Situation	Mental Set Slogan
Studying for an examination	"I am going to be relaxed and learn."
Running a race	"I am going to run fast and loose."
Asking for a date with a special person	"I am going to be happy, interesting,poised, and thoughtful."
Ringing doorbell on first date	"I am going to do everything possible to make this person happy."
In a crisis situation	"Stay calm. I will beat this. Stay calm."
Giving a speech	"I am going to be cool, poised, and humorous."

Bud Winters, *Relax and Win-Champion Performance in Whatever You Do*, p. 50-51.

Table 10.1

Yoga is nonsectarian.
It is a wise and prudent way of
going about life-it's a mental, spiritual,
and physical discipline. I have a good feeling
about myself when I'm doing it.
I get in touch with my whole body.

. . . **Kareem Abdul-Jabbar**

GENERAL SPORTS WARM-UP AND COOL-DOWN

Using yoga poses as a warm up and cool down routine for athletic activity can help prevent injuries. The yoga poses are done without bouncing or force and are executed in a slow relaxing manner as you concentrate on what the body is feeling. This development of concentration leads to a greater awareness of the body's movement and can carry over to the enhanced execution of the sports skill. Table 10.2 is a list of yoga poses that function as a general warm-up and cool down routine. In addition to these following poses, add those listed under the sport heading that is of interest to you.

General Sports Warm-Up and Cool-Down

Neck Turns (Fig. 3.2)	Neck Stretches (Fig. 3.1)
Body Rolls (Fig. 3.3)	Wall Stretch (Fig. 3.7)
Head of Cow (Fig. 10.6)	Chest Expansion (Fig. 10.1)
Tree (Fig. 3.28)	Spinal Twist (Fig. 10.2)
Dog (Fig. 10.7)	Locust-1/2 (Fig. 3.15)
Full Locust (Fig. 4.4)	Alternate Leg Stretch (Fig. 10.8)
Sitting Forward Bend (Fig. 10.5)	Sun Salute Routine (Fig. 4.20)
Moon Salute Routine (Fig. 3.35)	

Table 10.2

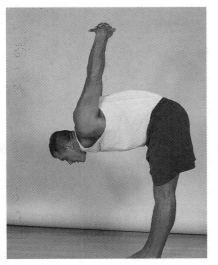

Figure 10.1   *Chest Expansion - Swimmer*

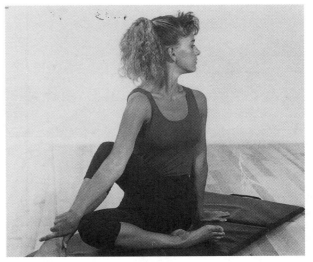

Figure 10.2   *Spinal Twist - Gymnast*

Racket Sports

Lunge (Fig. 4.1 on page 47)
Balance Posture (Fig. 4.9 on page 53)
Feldenkrais Kneeovers (Fig. 3.10 on page 19)
Warriors I, II & III (Figs. 4.14, 4.15 & 4.16 on
on pages 56, 57 & 58)

Running/Walking

Toe Hold Leg Lift (Fig. 10.4)
Feldenkrais Kneeovers (Fig. 3.10 on page 19)
Abdominal Lift (Fig. 3.31 on page 40)
Balance Posture (Fig. 4.9 on page 53)

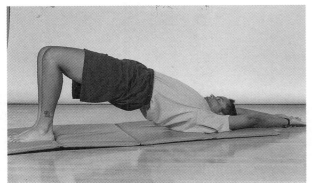

Figure 10.3   *Back Push-Up - Softball Player*

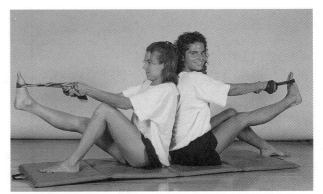

Figure 10.4   *Toe Hold Leg Lift - Track Athletes*

Volleyball

Lunge (Fig. 4.1 on page 47)
Abdominal Lift (Fig. 3.31 on page 40)
Feldenkrais Kneeovers (Fig. 3.10 on page 19)
Back push up (Fig. 10.3)
Cobra (Figs. 3.14A & B on page 22)
Warriors I, II, & III (Figs. 4.14, 4.15 & 4.16 on pages 56, 57 & 58)

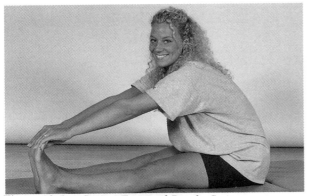

Figure 10.5   *Sitting Forward Bend - Swimmer*

Golf

Balance Posture (Fig. 4.9 on page 53)
Cobra (Figs. 3.14 A&B on page 22)

Weight Lifting

Toe Hold Leg Lift (Fig 10.4)
Balance Posture (Fig. 4.9 on page 53)
Abdominal Lift (Fig. 3.31 on page 40)
Cobra (Figs. 3.14 A&B on page 22)

Basketball

In 1961 Kareem Abdul-Jabbar discovered yoga and continued his stretching throughout his twenty-plus years playing basketball. He sees yoga as preventive maintenance which reduced his pulled muscles and other injuries. He has been interviewed in several magazines and always attributes his on-court success to hatha yoga. Since his retirement from the professional basketball scene he has continued his yoga practice with five classes a week.

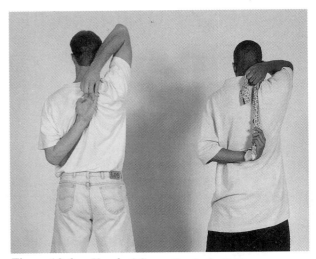

Figure 10.6   *Head of Cow - Basketball Player*

Basketball Poses

Lunge (Fig. 4.1 on page 47)
Abdominal Lift (Fig. 3.31 on page 40)
Feldenkrais Kneeovers (Fig. 3.10 on page 19)
Cobra (Fig. 3.14 A&B on page 22)
Warriors I, II, & III (Figs. 4.14, 4.15 & 4.16 on pages 56, 57 & 58)

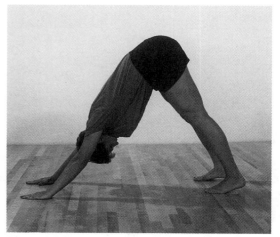

Figure 10.7   *Dog - Basketball Player*

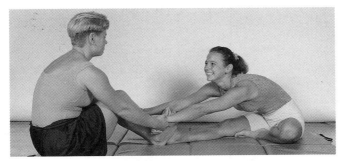

Figure 10.8   *Alternate Leg Stretch - Gymnasts*

Dance

Dancers have been using yoga poses for their stretching and warm up programs for years. You can capture a DANCE feeling when the hatha yoga routines, or postural flows such as the Sun and Moon Salute, are done to music. I enjoy doing the Sun Salute to the song "When Morning has Broken" by Cat Stevens. The style of yoga taught by Kali Ray is dance like in its style and in the feel that it gives to the participant.

The first series of Ashtanga yoga (Power Yoga) was the basis for a dance performance at the Dance Theatre Seven in Fairfax, CA. The performance was a balance betwen modern dance and the meditative quality of yoga asanas. Georgia Ortega, the choreographer of "Vision/Quest Journey" feels that she has only begun to tap into the possibilities of blending yoga and dance; not only for choreographic purposes but also for the benefits of strength, breath control and the awareness it offers to dancers.

SUMMARY

In addition to the above hatha yoga routines it is fun to do the partner routine (Fig. 4.23) as it can add to the feeling of teamwork and camaraderie between the members of a team. It is also fun to do some massage activities at the end of a practice (See Unit 11). Also remember that many athletes value the use of a flotation tank (Unit 6) and its positive influence on their sports performance through mental practice and release of stress. Continue on now by reading unit 11, " Other Ways to Body and Mind Awareness," for additional ideas on how yoga type activities can enhance your enjoyment and participation in sports and dance.

> *The Olympians show us what we're capable of in the moment of silence, the moment of truth—when we're called upon to go beyond the usual limits, into the realm of the warrior athlete. The word warrior conveys the concept which means one whose training develops, balances and integrates body, mind and emotions.*
> ... **Dan Millman**, *The Warrior Athlete*

RESOURCES

BOOKS

Birch, Beryl Bender. *Power Yoga.*   New York, N.Y. , Fireside , Simon & Shuster Publishing. 1995

Christensen, Alice. *The American Yoga Association Beginner's Manual.* New York, A Fireside Book, Simon & Schuster, Inc., 1987.

Couch, Jean and Weaver, Nell. *Runner's World Yoga Book.* Mountain View, CA. Runner's World Publications, Inc., 1979.

Folan, Lilias. *Lilias, Yoga, and Your Life.*   New York, Macmillan Publishing Co., Inc., l981.

Jackson, Ian Scott. *Yoga and the Athlete,* Mountain View, CA. World Publications, 1975.

Jois, Pattabhi, & Rosenthal, Ray. *Ashtanga Yoga, An Aerobic Yogic System.* Video cassette, cassette and instructional book. Hart Productions. 1989.

Kogler, Aladar. *Yoga for Every Athlete.*   Llewlen Publishers. 1990

Leonard, George. *Mastery.* New York, NY: Dutton/New American Library. 1990.

_____*The Ultimate Athlete: Revisioning Sports, Physical Education and the Body.*   Berkeley, CA. North Atlantic. 1990.

Millman, Dan. *The Way of the Peaceful Warrior.*   Los Angeles CA, J.P. Tarcher Publisher, 1980.

_____   *The Warrior Athlete : Body, Mind and Spirit.* Walpole, New Hampshire, Stillpoint Publishing. 1979.

_____ VIDEO *Peaceful Warrior Workout,* Sounds True Catalog. 735 Walnut St. Dept. SC8. Boulder, CO 80302.

Winter, Bud. *Relax and Win : Championship Performance In Whatever You Do.* San Diego, CA. A.S. Barnes and Company, Inc. 1981.

MAGAZINE ARTICLES

Barks, Joe and E.J. Muller. "Sports Yoga," *Men's Health.* February, 1993. p.48-51.

Cummins, Cynthia. "The Best-Kept Fitness Secret," *Women's Sports & Fitness.*   August/Sept. 1988. p. 50-52.

Festa, Susan A. "Body and Soul," *World Tennis,* November, 1989. p.65-67.

Fields, Rick. "Gentle Warrior," *Yoga Journal,* March/April, 1989. p 52-57,   105 & 107.

McNeill, Barbara. "Beyond Sports: Imaging in Daily Life," *Noetic Sciences Collection: 1980-1990 Ten Years of Consciousness Research.* Sausalito, CA Institute of Noetic Sciences. 1991 p. 32-34.

Rattenbury, Jeanne. "Yoga for Total Fitness," *Vegetarian Times.* September. 1993. p. 67-71.

Ries, Richard. "Try Yoga," *Bicycling.* December 1992, p. 66-67.

Rhodes, M. "Complimentary Exercise," *Women's Sports and Fitness.* January/February 1995, p. 45-50.

Wages, Joan. "Yoga + Football : A Winning Combination," *Yoga Journal,* November/December, l981, p.6-12.

Whitten, Philip. "The Joys of Mastery - Interview with George Leonard," *New Age Journal.* May/June 1990. p. 36-41, 114-118.

Other Ways to Body-Mind Awareness

> *If of thy mortal goods thou are bereft,*
> *And from thy slender store two loaves alone to thee are left,*
> *Sell one, and with the dole-*
> *Buy hyacinths to feed thy soul.*
>
> **. . . Mohammedan Sheik (1183 -1206)**

As your practice with yoga grows you become more aware of: 1. the connectedness of your whole self; 2. how you function; 3. an awareness of your postural habits; and 4. how you move. This unit will present basic information about other approaches to body/mind integration and alignment. Some of these "body therapies" were developed by people who did yoga and meditation. Each approach will be briefly described, and in the resource section under each heading there will be a listing of articles, books, audio tapes and the address of where to write for more information and the names of teachers or practioners who are trained and/or certified. I have personally experienced and enjoyed all of these approaches discussed in this unit.

ACUPUNCTURE AND ACUPRESSURE

Acupuncture and acupressure, two Chinese forms of healing that are over two thousand years old, are based on the principle of balance and harmony. There is a life-force energy running through our bodies which the Chinese call *chi* or *Qi* (called prana in yoga, see unit 5). This energy should run freely along pathways of energy called meridians. Along these fourteen meridians are nearly 400 sites, the acupuncture and acupressure points, where needles are inserted or pressure applied to help the energy run smoothly. The belief is that if there is an imbalance of energy then a person will experience symptoms of disease.

The diagnosis of a patient is very specific and based on asking many questions, looking and listening. Chinese medicine is very closely tied to nature and it is often believed that imbalances of the body arise from overexposure to cold, hot, damp or wind.

There are two aspects of chi, and these are **YIN** and **YANG**. The two energies have opposing qualities that must be in balance and work together for the body to be healthy. Table 11.1 below shows qualities of yin and yang.

YIN	YANG
Feminine	Masculine
Night	Day
Lower	Upper
Back	Front
Soft	Hard
Contracting	Expanding
Negative	Positive
Deficiency	Excess
Cold	Hot

Table 11.1

What does a typical acupuncture/accupressure treatment consist of? After the practioner has assessed the health situation and determined what needs to be treated, the sites on the meridians are chosen and wiped with an alcohol saturated cotton ball. The stainless steel needles are pre-sterilized, individually packaged and are disposable to prevent the transmission of infections. The needles are inserted to a depth of 1/4 to 1". The needles range in circumference from as thin as a hair to the largest, which is smaller than a sewing needle. They also are of varying lengthes with the longest needles being used on a large person who has a considerable layer of fat. The feeling as a needle is inserted is much milder than when you prick your finger with a pin. Blood is seldom drawn. When the needle is on the site and is gently moved by the practioner you will feel a tingling or an electric sensation similar to when you hit your elbows "crazy bone"- but it is a milder response. The number and frequency of accupuncture treatments varies and will be determined by the practioner and based on each individuals condition. Acupuncture treatments can be obtained in twenty-five states at present and the number is increasing yearly.

When choosing an acupuncturist you should refer to the following suggestions. After having passed an examination, acupuncturists are licensed either by the state in which they practice, or by the National Commission for the Certification of Acupuncturists (NCCA). You should also check their training and verify that their school was licensed. Are they board certified? And of extreme importance - recommendations from satisfied clients who have been helped by an acupuncture treatment.

Refer to Table 11.2 for a listing from the World Health Organization of what problems can be treated by acupuncture.

You can use pressure on acupuncture sites to help restore the balance of energy in the body. In the following diagrams (Fig. 11.1-.3) there are some acupuncture sites you can use to help yourself, or have a partner assist you in locating them. Remember that it is important to use fairly strong, evenly applied pressure on both sides of the body for a bilateral point, and to press for two to three minutes, then move to another site, or wait a few minutes and repeat the pressure.

1. Ear, Nose, and Throat Disorders: toothache, pain after tooth extraction, gingivitis, acute sinusitis, acute rhinitis, nasal catarrh and acute tonsillitis
2. Respiratory Disorders: bronchial asthma (when uncomplicated)
3. Gastrointestinal Disorders: esophageal and cardio spasm, hiccup, gastroptosis, gastritis, chronic duodenal ulcers, colonitis, vacillary dysentery, constipation, diarrhea and paralytic ileus
4. Eye Disorders: conjunctivitis, central retinitis, nearsightedness in children, and cataracts without complication
5. Neurological and Muscular Disorders: headaches, migraines, trigeminal neuralgia, facial paralysis within the first 3-6 months, post-stroke paresis, peripheral neuritis, neurological bladder dysfunction, bed wetting, intercostal neuralgia, cervical syndrome, frozen shoulder, tennis elbow, sciatica, low back pain, osteoarthritis, knee pain, sprains and strains and most gynecological complaints.

Table 11.2   *World Health Organization Acupuncture Treatment List*

Instructions for Locating Acupressure Sites (Front)

1. **Concentration, Memory Point**: Located on a line straight up from the nose, over the top of the head in a hollow just behind the crown

2. **Nasal Congestion Point**: Run finger up the side of the nose until it reaches the top of a triangle of cartilage

3. **Toothache Point**: Located in the corner of the jaw and found by running finger up towards ear (approximately 1 inch) until it falls in hollow

4. **Cough and Asthma Points** : 2 points: The first is located just over and behind the bone in the hollow of the throat. The second point is on the midline of the body even with the level of the nipples

5. **Stomach Ache Point**: Located on the midline of the front of the body halfway between the bottom of the sternum and the navel

6. **Water Retention and Menstrual Pain/Problems:** Located on the line going down the leg from the medial side of the kneecap, approximately 5 fingers distance from the kneecap and over the round top of the bone

7. **Water Retention and Menstrual Pain/Problems:** Located up from the inside of the ankle bone 4 fingers distance and back fron the shinbone approximately 1/2 to 3/4 inch

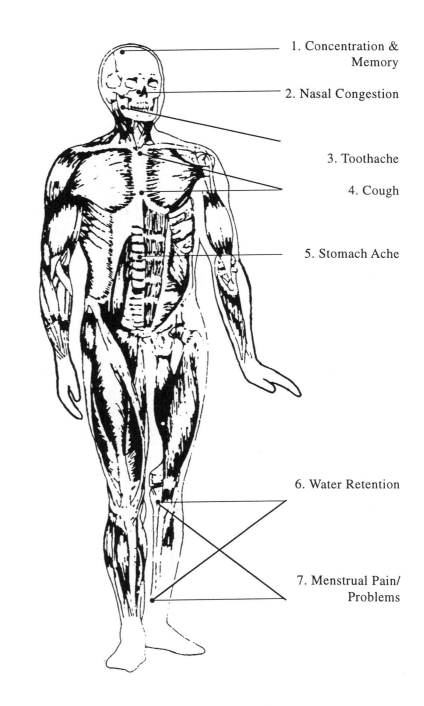

1. Concentration & Memory

2. Nasal Congestion

3. Toothache

4. Cough

5. Stomach Ache

6. Water Retention

7. Menstrual Pain/ Problems

Figure 11.1

Instructions for Locating Acupressure Sites (Back)

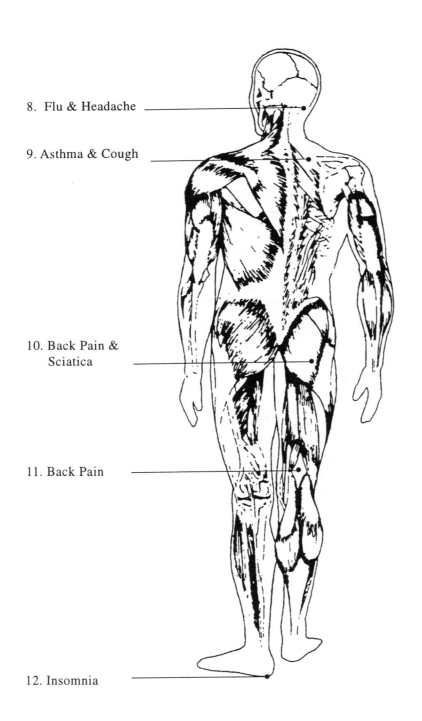

8. Flu & Headache

9. Asthma & Cough

10. Back Pain & Sciatica

11. Back Pain

12. Insomnia

8 . **Flu and Headache Point**: Located in a hollow where the skull meets the neck muscles on the back of the head. This point will be very sore if you are coming down with the flu or a cold

9. **Asthma and Cough Points** (3 points each side): Located approximately 1 inch, 1 1/2 inch and 2 inches out from the 1st thoracic vertebrae which is at the level of the shoulders

10. **Back Pain and Sciatica Point**: Located just lateral to the center of each buttock. You will be able to tell when you have located this point because it gives a strong reaction

11. **Back Pain Point**: Located on the crease in the center of the back of the knee and is easiest to find and apply pressure to while the knee is bent

12. **Insomnia Point**: In the center of the heel on the bottom of the foot

Figure 11.2

Instructions for Locating Acupressure Sites

13. **Insomnia Point**: Located just over the bone on crease of the wrist on a line running straight up the arm from the little finger

14. **Nausea, Morning and Carsickness Point**: Located on the inside of the wrist between the middle tendons and up the distance found by placing 4 fingers close together on the wrist crease

15. **Nosebleed Point**: Located on the outside corner of thumbnail. It is most effective to hold a burning stick of incense near the site to stop bleeding

16. **Headache and Toothache Point**: Located at the top of the fleshy mound found by bringing thumb next to hand . Press down on the top of the crease nearest wrist, and inward towards the fingers, while index finger is pressing up from the bottom. This gives a strong reaction

17. **Hiccups Point**: Located on the ear where the top part curves in and flattens out

18. **Headache, Hangover Point**: Located on the ear lobe

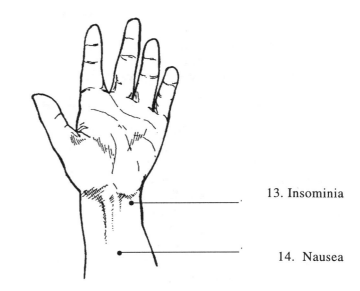

13. Insominia

14. Nausea

15. Nosebleed

16. Headache & Toothache

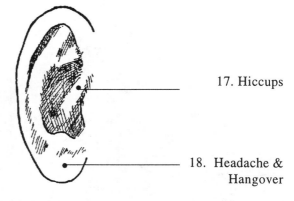

17. Hiccups

18. Headache & Hangover

Information by Rebecca Birkel, Dipl.Ac. New England School of Acupuncture, Boston, MA.
Drawings by Lydia Gerbig, a Ball State University graduate.

Figure 11.3

ALEXANDER TECHNIQUE

> *The Technique of F.M. Alexander may be described as a system for the proper use of the self, a method for the creative, conscious control of the whole psycho-physical organism*
> . . . **Aldous Huxley**

This technique was developed in 1900 by F.M. Alexander, an actor who was born in Tasmania. He developed a problem with hoarseness of his voice which could not be explained by the medical community. In an attempt to find a cause Alexander placed mirrors around his London flat to observe himself and eventually discovered that he threw his head back when speaking. This inhibited the flow of energy to his vocal chords and affected his speech. Out of this discovery he developed a system of observation by the self and by an Alexander teacher who would then help change the client's bad movement and alignment habits as observed in their daily activities. Several prominent men of the day; such as playright George Bernard Shaw, author Aldous Huxley, and educator John Dewey, were among those who learned and practiced the Alexander technique.

In this technique a person works with you giving you directions and gently touching you where you need a correction. A session lasts from 30-60 minutes. This technique is very popular with musicians and actors and is taught in many schools of music and theater around the world. The outcome is that a person becomes "educated" about how the performance of daily habits of movement can be changed to be done with less tension, increased lightness and fluidity, and enhanced poise. Following in Fig. 11.4, two yoga students are gently working with the alignment of the neck and shoulders.

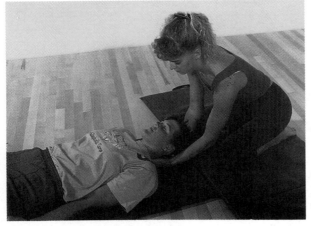

Figure 11.4   *Two Students Gently Working with Alignment*

AYURVEDA

> *Ayurveda seems to have remarkable results with many health problems Western medicine just can't touch.*
> **March/April 1994, *Yoga Journal***

Ayurvedic medicine developed in India at least 3000 years ago and is based on the concept that the body has the ability to heal itself. It is recognized as the FIRST organized approach to health developed on this planet that is based on the body itself and not on magic, supersition or spiritual forces. The word *Ayur* means life span and *veda* means knowledge or science. At the base of this ancient practice is the concept that when the body is out of harmony, disease will develop. This balance is based on three basic life forces or *doshas*- elements that exist in the environment and in the body.

> 1. VATA- air; produces movement
> 2. KAPHA- earth; stabilizes, body structure
> 3. PITTA- fire; heat, dehydration, digestion and the force that interfaces between the kapha and vata

There is a mixture of all three of these elements in a person, with one being the dominant resulting in body types, temperaments and chronic disorders. Example: a PITTA type would be described as being "fiery," passionate and could have rashs, heartburn or peptic ulcers. Patients are given questionnaires that aid in defining their dosha type. The Ayurvedic physician then gives them a physical exam that assesses their body's tissues (*dhatus),* and passageways of cleansing and elimination (*strotases).* The pulse is assessed in each wrist for pace, strength, pattern of movement (light or pounding) and how deep the three fingers can detect the pulse as it is connected to different organs. After the diagnosis, a treatment is prescribed which may involve adjusting the diet, taking herbal remedies, or using massages and steam treatments. In the United States, Ayurvedic medicine is not licensed and those who are trained in it are also accredited as a physician, chiropractor, nutritionist or another health-care practicioner. In India the physicians educated in Ayurvedic medicine complete a five and a half year program of study and residency. For more information about Ayurveda refer to the best-sellers written by Deepak Chopra, M.D., and Vassant Lad, M.D. ,that are listed in the resources. You can also locate the name of an Ayurvedic physician in your area trained by Maharishi Ayur-Veda, by referring to the resources for the telephone number of the spa *The Raj* .

CHIROPRACTIC

> *Look well to the spine*
> *for the cause of disease.*
> ... Hippocrates, 4th Century B.C., Greece.

The word "chiropractic" comes from a Greek word for manual medicine. Dexter Nardella, D.C. explains the practice of chiropractic as being a clinical science which is based upon: 1. the law of biology which states that there is a capacity in all living things to be well (Homeostasis); 2. the theory of physiology that the nervous system provides total control of the body's functions; 3. the chiropractic hypothesis that health in the nervous system relates to health in the body; and 4. the <u>major</u> premise of chiropractic- there is a relationship between the framework of the spine and the health of the nervous system.

The art of chiropractic lies in the use of the hands to detect minute changes in spinal function and to correct those changes using refined techniques of spinal adjustment or manipulation.

Chiropractic's success with a variety of diseases is well documented. And yet its purpose in caring for people is not to treat disease. The purpose of the chiropractor is to correct nerve interference from the spine (vertebral subluxation). You might say that chiropractors care for the well-being of the entire person who has the disease rather than only treating a specific disease.

Chiropractic is now making a contribution to the Sports Medicine scene as it is now a component of the United States Olympic Committee's Medical Staff, primarily at the request of the athletes. Greg Louganis, winner of two gold medals in diving, struck his head on the platform during competition, and following a spinal adjustment by a chiropractor he returned to win his third gold medal in the 1984 Seoul Olympics. Chiropractic is also being used as a therapy or treatment for: athletes from the football teams of Miami Dolphins, San Francisco 49ers; the competitors at the 1987 Pan American Games in Indianapolis; the 1988 United States Greco-Roman Wrestling team; individual athletes such as Bruce Jenner, Suzy Chaffee, Francie Larrieu, Henry Rono, and Dwight Stone. The use of a chiropracter as a "team doctor" for elementary children to the Olympic level athletes has been growing in popularity. "Weekend athletes" can also benefit from a visit to a chiropractor.

FELDENKRAIS METHOD

> *The body can only do*
> *what the nervous system makes it do.*
> ... Moshe Feldenkrais

This approach to body work was developed by Moshe Feldenkrais, Ph. D., in the 1940s. Russian by birth, educated as a physicist, and a mechanical and electrical engineer with a science doctorate from the Sorbonne, he became interested in the body's mechanics. He was a European champion in Judo holding a black belt and had spent time in India studying yoga. His growing interest in body movement expanded when an old soccer injury to his knee became a problem. He then began studying ways to help himself. Out of this study and interest evolved his two teaching methods; 1. "Functional Integration" (FI), which is hands on work practiced one to one; and 2. "Awareness Through Movement" (ATM), which consists of simple movement exercises which are usually taught in a class. Reports of his work led people to Israel to be trained by him and to his also becoming an author.

The basis for this body work is to use simple, non-habitual movement and to link this movement with the nervous system and the ways we learn. Developing a new movement pattern can stimulate the brain and break old harmful habits of movement and alignment (see Fig. 11.5A&B). His methods have been researched and are now taught by over 300 practitioners worldwide. His program of movement has been taught to those with cerebral palsy, brain and spinal cord injuries as well as famous people such as "Dr. J." Julius Erving of basketball fame, violinist Yehudi Menuhin, anthropologist Margaret Mead and film director Peter Brook. Feldenkrais always emphasized that his technique did not "cure," but that if a person had trouble with movement he could probably improve the movement and thereby improve their health and well being.

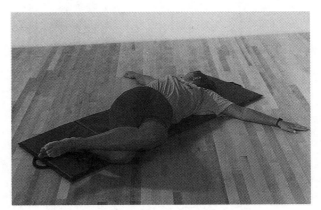

Figure 11.5A   *Feldenkrais Kneeovers*

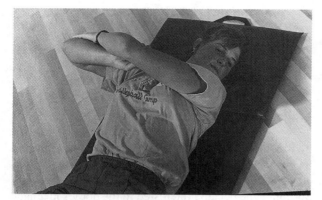

Figure 11.5B *Feldenkrais Arms*

MASSAGE THERAPY

The technique of massage is directed toward working with the muscles and joints of the body to relieve tension and improve alignment and circulation. Those trained as a massage therapist have studied anatomy and physiology as well as a variety of massage techniques such as Swedish, Shiatsu, and Reflexology.

It is very helpful if you are recovering from an injury or have a chronic alignment problem caused by scoliosis, for example. The American Association of Massage Therapists maintains a list of those certified to practice.

It is becoming popular to use some massage techniques along with the counterposes in yoga classes to help alleviate muscle tension (Fig. 11.6).

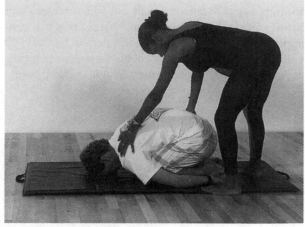

Figure 11.6   *Back Stretch*

A tip I learned from my massage therapist that also relieves muscle tension is to soak for 30 minutes in a bath tub of hot water to which you have added one quart of apple cider vinegar (not the syn-

thetic type). She recommends to all her clients to do this following their visit to her as this alleviates the muscle soreness that comes from increasing the circulation and affecting the position and alignment of the body parts. A chemistry student in one of my yoga classes explained why this is effective- "Most vinegars are a hydrogen gased, positively charged ion bonded covalently to a negaively charged hydroxide ion, ON-. The hydroxide ion (-1.6 x 10-19 coulombs) is basic and may through absorption, negate the soreness of muscles through overuse by combining with the positive ion from lactic acid." Try this bath if you have been inactive for a while and over did in any form of exercising such as the first day back in an aerobics dance class or the first few days of athletic practice.

TRAGER WORK

> *What I really get out of this work is to feel the response of tissue in the person. To feel it actualy come up into your hands, feel the change in the body, see the change in the face.*
>   . . . **Milton Trager M.D.**

Milton Trager M.D., was born in Chicago and at sixteen moved to Miami where he trained as a boxer. He developed an interest in working with the body and helping people in his neighborhood and on Miami Beach with their aches and pains. In 1941 he received a Doctorate of Physical Medicine from the Los Angeles College of Drugless Physicians and during World War II he worked in the Physical Therapy Departmemt of the Navy. At the age of forty-one he tried to get admitted to American medical schools but all seventy that he applied to turned him down as they thought he was to old. He was accepted into Universitarie Autonoma de Guadalajara in Mexico, where they organized a clinic for him to treat polio victims. He received his medical degree in 1955 and went to Hawaii. Here he met Maharishi Mahesh Yogi and became interested in Transcendental Meditation. People heard of his body work and many of those he had helped encouraged him to teach his method to others. Finally, in 1977, he closed his private medical practice in Honolulu, and founded the Trager Institute located in Mill Valley, California. There are now well over 2000 Trager students throughout the world and more than 300 practitioners. To locate one, see the resource section for the address

The Trager method, like that of Feldenkrais, has two basic approaches. In the first appproach the practioner works with the client on a massage table.

This is called "Trager Psychophysical Integration" (TPI), and consists of a gentle rolling, rocking, and wiggling of the body (See Fig. 11.7). The practitioner does what is referred to as "hook up" which is to connect with the client in a gentle "meditation in motion" style. The experience of TPI is very relaxing as the touch is very light and feathery and never forceful. The goal is to help allow the mind to help the body to release the tension - not increase the tension by attacking it and maybe causing discomfort.

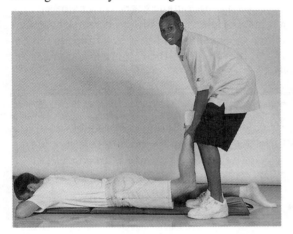

Figure 11.7 *Basketball Players Doing Tragering*

The second approach is known as "Mentastics," a word coined by Dr. Trager from "mental gymnastics." This activity is done in a class with a teacher leading you through some shaking and loosening types of exercise. You use the motion in the tissue, muscles and joints to produce a sensory feeling that will enter the central nervous system and start the mind connecting to the muscles in a new sensory-motor pattern. The hope is that the body will feel lighter and then will stand and move lighter resulting in a new ease in how daily activities are performed.

The Trager method has been of help to many afflicted with polio, muscular dystrophy, multiple sclerosis as well as those with old injuries and body alignment problems.

I teach my students how to be spontaneous and spirited within the Tai Ji form, so they can choose any choreography they wish to dance in, especially their own.

. . . Chung Liang Al Huang,
Embrace Tiger
Return to Mountain

TAI JI CHUAN/QI GONG

..estimates suggest that 50-60 million Chinese practice Qi Gong at dawn each day for the purpose of disease prevention or in an attempt to alter the natural course of serious or lethal illness.
. . . David Eisenberg M.D.,
Harvard Medical School

Tai Ji Chuan is almost as old as yoga and it is also based on the theory of life force, which in China is referred to as "Chi" or "Qi." Tai Ji is a series of poses that are connected into routines of varying lengths. Popular here in the United States is the Twenty-Four Step routine. The theory of Yin and Yang, discussed in the acupuncture section, is a concept that is also present in the practice of Tai Ji.

Tai Ji is done in a slow manner with a very controlled, smooth style that looks effortless but is not as the body is controlled and moved with energy and awareness (see Fig 11.8). The use of the breath and balance are important components as well. It can improve posture, flexibility, muscular strength, balance, breath control, concentration andcan also lower stress. Once Tai Ji is learned it can be practiced for the rest of one's life with no expense - just like yoga can be done.

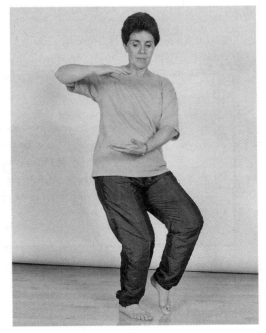

Figure 11.8 *Author Demonstrating Tai Ji Chuan*

FURTHER STUDY

> *Be more concerned that I'm always learning*
> *than that I'm always teaching*
> . . . **Lee J. Painter,**
> *If Forever Came Tomorrow*

There are many opportunities for enhancing your interest in yoga and other mind/body techniques and furthering your education. Many of the teachers mentioned in this book offer teacher training sessions of varying lengths from a weekend to several months. They are often advertised in the *Yoga Journal* and the *Yoga International* magazines. As an example of these offerings there is the "Yoga With Heart" -adapting Yoga for Heart Disease, held in 1995 in California. This program was taught by Judith Lasater, Ph.D. and two of the instructors who are a part of Dr. Dean Ornish's Program for Reversing Heart Disease, Nischala Joy Devi director of the Stress Management Program, and Amy Kline-Gage who is the yoga teacher that works with the research participants..

Attending other conferences, such as the ones sponsored by the Association for Humanistic Psychology, is also a possibility. Sonoma State University, Sonoma CA, along with Integrative Yoga Therapy, Mill Valley, CA, is now offering a Masters Degree in Psychology with a focus in Yoga and Mind-Body Health. They also offer a variety of two week training programs throughout the year. The Feathered Pipe Foundation, in Helena, MT, offers one week programs throughout the summer and also yoga trips to the Bahamas and Mexico. See the resource section for addresses.

> *They have classes for learning how to play*
> *tennis, and courses on how to write books,*
> *but where do I sign up to learn how to live life?*
> . . . **Anne Wilson Schaef**

SUMMARY

If you are enjoying Hatha Yoga and like this approach to exercise you will probably enjoy doing any of the above programs also. These are all approaches that can be practiced throughout a person's lifespan.

I would like to end this book by sharing with you Ram Dass' interpretation of the traditional greeting of India, "Namaste," from his book *Grist for the Mill*.

> *Namaste*
>
> *"In India when we meet and part we often say, 'NAMASTE,' which means*
> *I honor the place in you where the entire universe resides,*
> *I honor the place in you of love, of light, of peace.*
> *I honor the place within you where if you are in that place in you*
> *and I am in that place in me, there is only one of us."*
>
> **Ram Dass,** *Grist for the Mill.*

RESOURCES

Batson, Glenna. "Dancing Fully, Safely, and Expressively- The Role of the Body Therapies in Dance Training," *Journal of Physical Education Recreation and Dance* . November/ December. 1990. p. 28-31.

Thompson, Keith. "The Future of The Body," *Yoga Journal,* May/June 1989, p.38-45,97.

Acupuncture

Traditional Acupuncture Foundation, American City Building, Columbia MD. 21044.Acupuncture Research Insti tute, 313 W. Andrix St., Monterey Park, CA. 91754.

Brady, Sally R. "Acupuncture and Me," *Good Housekeeping.* August 1987, p. 58, 60-62.

Eisenberg, David M.D. "Energy Medicine In China: Defining a Research Strategy Which Embraces the Criticism of Skeptical Colleagues," *Noetic Sciences Collection: 1980-1990 Ten Years of Consciousness Research.*

Sausalito, CA: The Institute of Noetic Sciences. 1991. p. 94-101.

Firebruce, Peter & Hill, Sandra. *Acupuncture; How it Works, How it Cures.* New Canaan, CT: Keats Publishing Inc. 1994.

Nickel, David J. *Acupressure for Athletes.* Santa Monica CA: Health Acu Press. 1984.

Rodarmor, William. "Acupuncture Comes of Age in America," *Yoga Journal.* March/April 1986. p. 26-29, 64.

Stein, Douglas. "Interview with Ji-Sheng Han," *Omni Magazine.* Feb. 1988, p. 81-2, 84-5, 102-3.

Wagner, Lindsay and Robt. M Klein. "The Acupressure Face-Lift," *New Age Journal.* March/April, 1989 p. 29-34.

Wilson, Beth. "Acupuncture: Healing More Than Pain," *Changing Woman.* Summer 1988, p. 17-18.

Alexander Technique

Alexander, F. Matthias. *Man's Supreme Inheritance.* London: Chaterson, 1946.

_____ *The Use of the Self.* London: Re-Educational Publications, 1955.

_____*Alexander Technique.* London: Thames and Hudson, 1974.

Barker, Sarah. *The Alexander Technique.* New York: Bantam, 1978.

Barlow, Wilfred. *The Alexander Principle.* New York; Random House, 1973.

American Center for Alexander Technique, Abraham Goodman House, 1 W. 67th St. New York NY (212) 799-0468.

The Society of Teachers of The Alexander Technique, 3b Albert Court, Kensington Gore,

London SW 7, England. Telephone 01-589-3834.

Ayurveda

Chopra, Deepak, M.D. *Ageless Body, Timeless Mind* . New York, NY: Harmony Books. 1993.

Chopra, Deepak, M.D. *Quantum Healing: Toward Perfect Health.* New York, NY: Bantam. 1990

_____ *Perfect Health: The Complete Mind/Body Guide.* New York, NY: Harmony Books.1991.

Lad, Vasant M.D. *Ayurveda: The Science of Life* . Six Audio cassettes with booklet. Sounds True Catalog, 735 Walnut St. Dept SC8, Boulder, CO. 1-800-333-9185.

_____ *Ayurveda, The Science of Selff-Healing: A Practical Guide.* Twin Lakes, WI. Lotus Light. 1991.

Herriott, Eva. "Staying Healthy with Ayurveda," *Yoga Journal.* March/April 1994 Issue 115. p. 84,86-92.

SPA- *The Raj,* Fairfield, IA. 1-800-248-9050.

Chiropractic

Haldeman, S. "Spinal Manipulative Therapy in Sports Medicine,"*Clinics in Sports Medicine* , 1986, p. 277.

Feldenkrais

Feldenkrais, Moshe. *Awareness Through Movement.* New York: Harper & Row, 1977.

_____. *The Elusive Obvious.* Cypertino, CA: Meta Publications, 1981.

Houston, Jean. *The Possible Human,* Los Angeles, CA: J. P. Tarcher, Inc., 1982.

Master, Robert and Jean Houston. *Listening to the Body.* New York, Delacorte Press, 1981.

Holmes, B. " Moving Well with Feldenkrais," *Yoga Journal,* Janurary/February, 1984, p. 30-32.

Rosenfeld, A. " Teaching the Body How to Program the Brain is Moshe's Miracle," *Smithsonian.* January 1981 Audio Tapes

Feldenkrais Guild. P.O. Box 11145, San Francisco, CA 94101.

Grotte, Josef Della Ph.D. P. O Box 612, Westminster MA. 01473.

Holmes, Bruce. 801 Madison Ave. Dept. J11, Evanston, IL 60202 (312) 869-3434.

Massage

James Bowling, Executive Secretary/Treasurer, American Massage and Therapy Association, P.O. Box 1270, 310 Cherokee St., Kingsport, TN 37660. Phone (615) 245-8071.
Inkeles, G., *The New Massage.* New York: Putnam 1980.
Montagu, Ashley, *Touching.* New York: Harper & Row, 1978.

Trager Method

Cavanaugh Carol, "The Work of Milton Trager," *The Yoga Journal.* September/October. 1982, p.20-25.
Drury Nevill, *The Bodywork Book,* Prism Alpha, P.O Box 778, San Leandro, CA 94577. 1984.
Griffin, Joe L. "How Trager Movement Education Improves Athletic Performance." *How Anybody Can Learn to Swim Well."* Silver Spring, MD. 1989.
Trager Institute, 300 Poplar Avenue, Suite #5, Mill Valley, CA 94941.

Tai Chi Chuan

Directory of Teachers- Tai Chi Association, P.O. Box 56113, Atlanta, GA: 30343.
Connor, Danny and Master Michael Tse. *Qi Gong.* York Beach, ME: Samuel Weiser, Inc. 1992.
Dunn Terrence. "The Practice and Spirit of Tai Chi Chuan". *Yoga Journal.* November/December, 1987.
Friedman, Milton."Chungliang Al Juang- A Master of Moving Meditatio,." *New Realities.* May/June 1989. p. 11-20.
Miller, Don and Julian."An Ancient Art Can Change Your Running," *Runner's World.* March 1982. p. 58-61, 89-90.
Perry, Paul. "Grasp The Bird's Tail," *American Health.* Janurary/February. 1986. p. 58-63.

Furthur Study

International Association of Yoga Therapists, Att. Diane. 3740 Sundale Road, Lafayette, Ca 94549. 510/284-3908.
Integrative Yoga Therapy, 305 Vista de Valle, Mill Valley CA 94941. 800/750-YOGA.
Feathered Pipe Foundation, P.O. Box 1682YI, Helena MT 59624. 406-442-8196.
Mind-Body Health Study Group Network of the Institute of Noetic Sciences, 444 North Capitol Street, Suite 428, Washington, D.C. 20001. 202/393-2208

APPENDICES

Stress Releases and Safety Valves

A

I do well	I'm average	Need to improve	
5	3	1	*(Place a check in the appropriate column. Try to be completely honest.*

_____ _____ _____ 1. "Owning" my own stress (not blaming others).

_____ _____ _____ 2. Knowing my level of optimum stress (the level of stress that allows you to do your best without becoming destructive).

_____ _____ _____ 3. Balancing work and play (scheduling time for play.)

_____ _____ _____ 4 Loafing more (learning to do nothing at times and feel okay about it).

_____ _____ _____ 5. Getting enough sleep and rest rather than ending up with what is left over at the end of the day (scheduling adequate sleep

_____ _____ _____ 7. Working off tension (hard physical effort on a regular basis).

_____ _____ _____ 8. Setting realistic goals (goals that can be acieved within a resonable time frame).

_____ _____ _____ 9. Practicing relaxation (meditating with music or biofeedback).

_____ _____ _____ 10. Slowing down (taking pleasure in every moment rather than rushing through life).

_____ _____ _____ 11. Putting emphasis on being rather than doing (being a person others like to be around is more important than "doing" many activities).

_____ _____ _____ 12. Managing my time, including planning for time alone (setting priorities and doing those things that are most important).

_____ _____ _____ 13. Planning regular recreation (recreation is a complete change of pace and something that is fun to do).

_____ _____ _____ 14. Having a physical fitness program (having a specific plan for strenuous exercise).

_____ _____ _____ 15. Avoiding too much caffeine (limiting coffee and cola drinks).

_____ _____ _____ 16. Emphasize good nutrition in diet (learning about nutrition and avoiding junk foods).

_____ _____ _____ 17. Avoiding alcohol or other chemicals to deal with pressure (dependency on alcohol or drugs deals with symptoms rather than the problem).

_____ _____ _____ 18. Avoiding emotional "overload (taking on problems of others when you are under stress is destructive).

_____ _____ _____ 19. Selecting emotional "investments" more carefully (of things we can get involved with that call for emotional involvement, it is necessary to choose carefully).

_____ _____ _____ 20. Giving and accepting positive "strokes" (being able to express positive things to others and receive positive comments in return is an achievement).

_____ _____ _____ 21. Talking out troubles and getting professional help if needed (being willing to seek help is a sign of strength rather than weakness).

Score Yourself

If you scored between 21 and 50, there are several areas you need to develop to better release your stress. It might be a good idea to discuss some of your answers with a counsellor or close friend.

If you scored between 51 and 75, you have discovered a variety of ways to deal efectively with stress. Make a note of those items you checked "need to improve" and work on strategies to helpyou move to the "I'm Average" box.

If you score was 75 or greater - congratulations. You apparently have found some excellent ways to deal with frustration and the complexities of life. Stay alert to protect the valuable skills you have acquired.

Reprinted with permission of Crisp Publications as it appears in *Mental Fitness: A Guide To Emotional Health*, by Merril F Raber, M.S.W., Ph. D. and George Dyck M.D., pages 23 &24.

B

Health History Questionnaire

NAME _____ AGE _____ STUDENT I.D.# _____

DATE OF LAST MEDICAL CHECKUP _____ PHONE _____

HOUR CLASS MEETS _____ YEAR IN SCHOOL _____ MAJOR _____

Please identify conditions that pertain to you.

_____ Heart problems

_____ Blood pressure

_____ Chest pain and discomfort

_____ Family history of
                 heart disease

_____ Allergies

_____ Asthmas

_____ Depression

_____ Diabetes

_____ Epilepsy

_____ Severe headaches

_____ Fainting

_____ Menstrual problems

_____ Pregnant

_____ Sleep disorders

_____ Smoking

_____ Drinking excessively

_____ Easting disorder

_____ Scoliosis

Injuries to:

_____ Foot

_____ Shoulder

_____ Cervical (Neck)

_____ Thoracic (Upper back)

_____ Lumbar (Lower back)

_____ Knees

_____ Ankles

Please list any other conditions that you think are important to bring to the attention of your instructor. _____

_____

Please list any medications that you take regularly. _____

C

Body Analysis Record Form

NAME _____ CLASS _____ SEC. _____

	START	MIDDLE	15TH WEEK
DATE	_____	_____	_____
RESTING PULSE	_____	_____	_____
WEIGHT	_____	_____	_____
HEIGHT	_____	_____	_____

GIRTH MEASUREMENTS: Standing - tape level, and refer to Unit 2 for complete instructions.

	START	MIDDLE	15TH WEEK
Chest-fullest	_____	_____	_____
Abdominal 1- over ribs	_____	_____	_____
Waist-narrowest	_____	_____	_____
Abdominal 2- over stomach	_____	_____	_____
Hips- over pubic bone	_____	_____	_____
Right Thigh- near crotch	_____	_____	_____
Right Calf- fullest	_____	_____	_____
Right Ankle- above bone	_____	_____	_____
Right Upper Arm- near armpit	_____	_____	_____
Right Wrist- below the bone	_____	_____	_____

WAIST TO HIP RATIO waist
*   (F- ↑ .8; M- ↑ .95)   **hip**

	START	MIDDLE	15TH WEEK
	_____	_____	_____
	_____	_____	_____

FLEXIBILITY

	START	MIDDLE	15TH WEEK
Sit and Reach (+ or - number)	_____	_____	_____
Hips	R ____ L ____	R ____ L ____	R ____ L ____
Shoulders	R ____ L ____	R ____ L ____	R ____ L ____
Trunk Lift	_____	_____	_____

D

Skeleton Front View

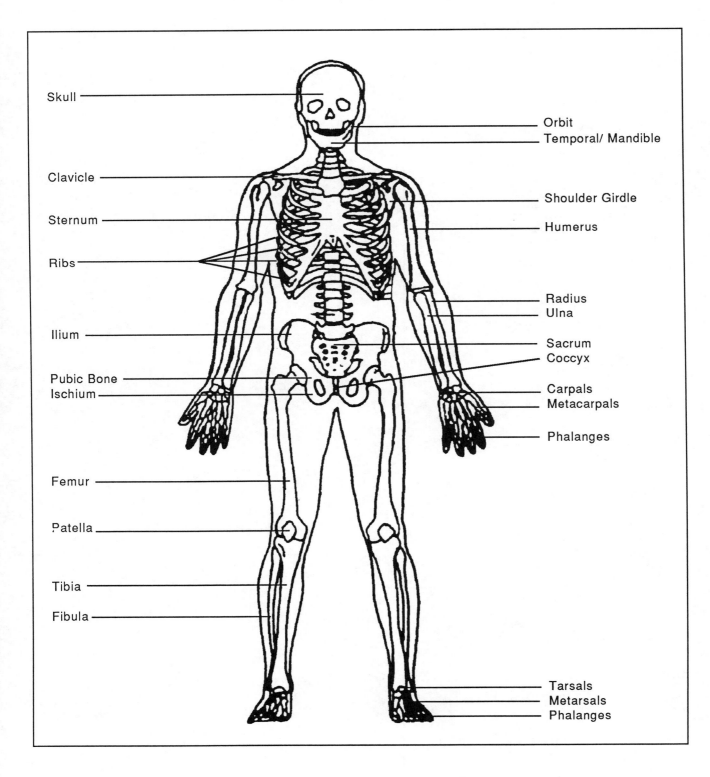

Skull

Clavicle

Sternum

Ribs

Ilium

Pubic Bone
Ischium

Femur

Patella

Tibia

Fibula

Orbit
Temporal/ Mandible

Shoulder Girdle

Humerus

Radius
Ulna

Sacrum
Coccyx

Carpals
Metacarpals

Phalanges

Tarsals
Metarsals
Phalanges

Skeleton Back View

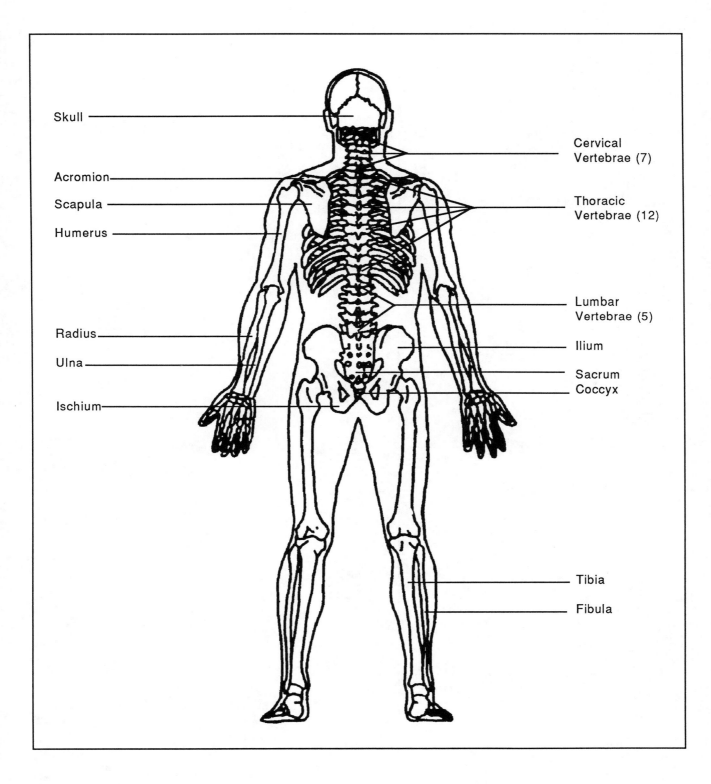

Skull

Acromion

Scapula

Humerus

Radius

Ulna

Ischium

Cervical
Vertebrae (7)

Thoracic
Vertebrae (12)

Lumbar
Vertebrae (5)

Ilium

Sacrum
Coccyx

Tibia

Fibula

Muscles Front View

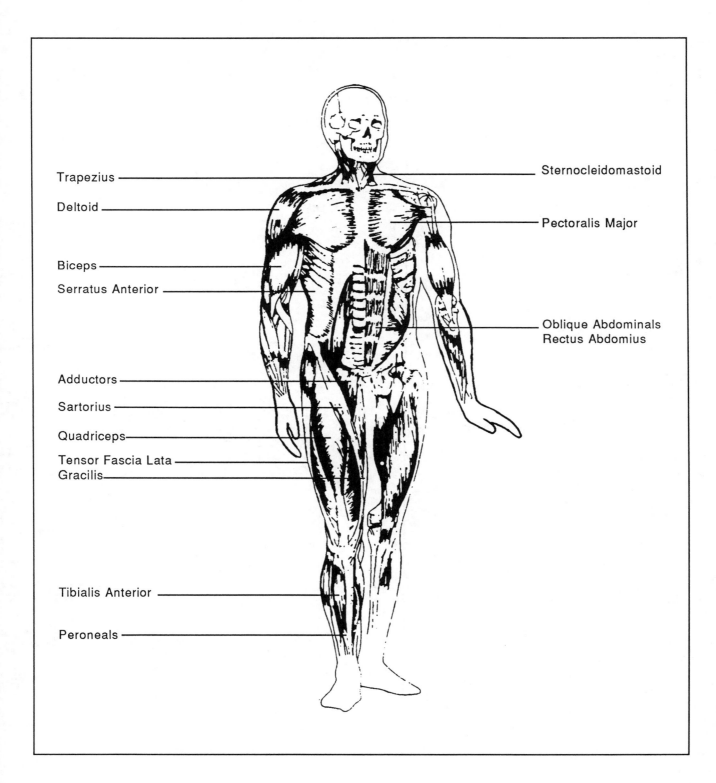

Trapezius ———————————————

Deltoid ————————————————

Biceps ——————————————

Serratus Anterior ——————————

Adductors ——————————

Sartorius ——————————

Quadriceps ——————————

Tensor Fascia Lata ——————————
Gracilis ——————————

Tibialis Anterior ——————————

Peroneals ——————————

——————————— Sternocleidomastoid

——————————— Pectoralis Major

——————————— Oblique Abdominals
Rectus Abdomius

Muscles Back View

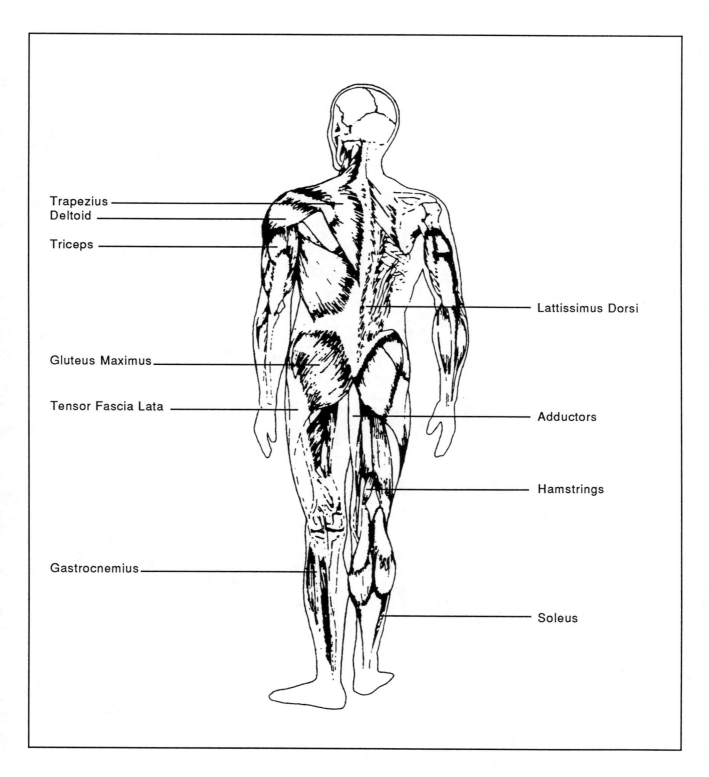

Trapezius

Deltoid

Triceps

Gluteus Maximus

Tensor Fascia Lata

Gastrocnemius

Lattissimus Dorsi

Adductors

Hamstrings

Soleus

F

RECIPES

Oat and Wheat Pancakes

You can mix this easy batter up to 18 hours ahead. Refrigerate, then stir before using. Makes 12 pancakes.1 1/4 cups oats and 2 cups skim milk- mix and let stand 10 mins. Stir in 1 egg, 1/2 cup all-purpose flour, 1/4 cup toasted wheat germ, 1 Tb. sugar, 1Tb. baking powder, 2 tsp. vegetable oil and 1/2 tsp salt. For each pancake pour a scant 1/4 cup of batter on hot well-greased griddle over medium-low heat. Cook turning once, until well browned on both sides and cooked through.
Per pancake; 92 cal, 4 g pro, 14, g car, 2 g fat, 22 mg chol, 201 mg sod.

Nebraska Bran Muffins

from Diet for a Small Planet, Frances Moore Lappe', p. 325, Ballantine Books, NY. 1979.
In a large bowl mix and let stand: 3 cups bran flakes (can substitue part All-Bran cereal) and 1 cup boiling water. Beat in medium bowl 2 eggs, 1 1/4 cup sugar or 1 cup honey, 2 cups buttermilk, 1/2 cup corn or other oil. Add to bran mixture. Sift together 2 cups whole wheat flour, 1/2 cup soy flour, 2 1/2 tsp soda, 1/2 tsp salt and fold into bran. Bake at 370° for 15 minutes in a greased muffin tin. A variation of these muffins was developed for the Nebraska Centennial in 1966. The addition of the soy is quite fitting and increases the protein content and usability. The batter may berefrigerated in covered jars several weeks. 2 muffins= approximately 6 g usable protein, 14-17% of daily protein allowance.

Irish Soda Bread (1994 First Prize)

This bread does not need any time to rise but it should sit about 6 hours after it comes out of the oven before it is sliced. If the crust seems too hard, wrap the baked bread in a damp tea towel and stand upright until it is cool. I like to bake this bread in a cast iron skillet with another skillet or an ovenproof lid to cover. This is more like the way it was originally made in Ireland over a peat fire in a fireplace.Mix 3 cups stone-ground whole-wheat flour, 1-1/2 cups white flour, 1/2 tsp salt, 1/2 tsp baking soda, 1 tsp cream of tartar or baking powder, 1 Tbl oat bran, 1 Tbl wheat germ and a handful of oatmeal. Make a well in the center and gradually mix in 1-1/2 cups buttermilk, sour milk or sweet milk, 1 egg, 1 Tbl sunflower oil and 1 Tbl honey. You may need less or more liquid-it depends on the absorbent quality of the flour. The dough should be soft and manageable. Knead dough into a ball in the mixing bowl with floured hands. Put in lightly floured skillet and flatten out till touching sides. Cut a deep cross with a floured knife through the center of the bread so it will easily break in quarters when it is baked. Bake at 400° for 25-30 minutes, check after 10 min, and if too brown, reduce the heat to 375°.

Birkel's Tabouli

Place 1 1/4 cup bulgur in bowl and cover with very hot water and let stand until light and fluffy. Drain of any excess water. Mix 1 cup minced, fresh mint, 2 cups minced parsley, 1 small cucumber seeded and chopped, 1 small onion chopped or 6 green topped onions, 1/2 green pepper, and 2 chopped tomatoes and add all to bulgur. DRESSING: 3/4 cup lemon juice, 1/4 cup (or less) olive oil, (optional) 1/2 tsp salt, and 1/2 tsp cumin. Chill and serve on a lettuce leaf.
Will not spoil like a cream type salad. Good for summer picnics. Serves 6-8.

Tomato-Basil Salad (Anti-Cancer)

Slice 4 medium tomatoes, and 1 small red onion thinly; Mix with 1/4 cup fresh basil (or 2 tsp. dried basil). Pour 1/4 -1/3 cup red wine vinegar over the salad and add   black pepper to taste. Let marinate at least 1/2 hour, preferably 1-2 hours. Serves 4-5.

Tofu Onion Garlic Dip

Combine all in a blender and mix until smooth: 1 lb. tofu, 1/4 c. oil, 3 Tbs. vinegar, 1 tsp. garlic powder (or real garlic minced), l medium onion, minced and 1 Tbs. soy sauce (if desired). Serve with crackers or fresh vegetables such16 as broccoli, celery, etc.

Tofu Cheesecake

Crust: Preheat oven to 350° In a 9" pie pan, melt 1/2 c. margarine add 1 package graham crackers crushed into fine crumbs. Bake 10 mins. and set aside.

Filling: Combine in a blender and mix until smooth: 24 oz. tofu(or 1 lb tofu and 8 oz. cream cheese), 2 eggs, 2/3 cup honey, (or 1/2 cup sugar), 1 Tbs. vanilla, 2 Tbs. vegetable oil, 1 Tbs. lemon juice, 1/8 tsp nutmeg, and 1/4 tsp. salt. Pour the filling into the crust and bake at 350 ' for 40 minutes (or until golden brown). Top with your favorite fruit or eat plain.

Pasta Primavera

2 servings

1/4 lb. whole-wheat noodles (fettuccine)
1/2 onion, chopped
1 clove elephant garlic, or 4-6 cloves regular garlic, finely chopped 1 tsp. olive oil
4-5 fresh mushrooms,
1/2 medium red bell pepper
1-2 plum tomatoes (Roma)
1/2 cup chopped parsley
1/4 to 1/2 cup spaghetti sauce
3 Tbs. salsa

Boil noodles for 10 minutes. While they are cooking saute onion and garlic in oil in nonstick skillet until onion is translucent. Add mushrooms and cook for 1 minute then add chopped pepper, tomato, parsley. Stir completely. Add spaghetti sauce and salsa and simmer 3-5 minutes until parsly is thoroughly cooked. In large bowl toss noodles with sauce. Sprinkle with parmesan cheese if desired.

Homemade Lowfat Yogurt

Soften 1/4 tsp gelatine and add boiling water to make 1 cup. Add 1/2 Tbl. sugar and cool. Mix 1 1/2 cup instant milk (dry powdered) with 1 1/2 cups water, add 1 small can evaporated milk and 1 more cup of tepid water and the gelatin mixture. Add 1 1/2 Tbl. of yogurt and stir thoroughly.

If you have a yogurt maker fill the jars and let them set for 10 hours. Or pour the mixture into clean glasses or small jars. Put the jars in a large pan of warm water. Cover the jars with clear plastic wrap. Place in a warm oven. Maintain the temperature of water between 100 ° and 120° F. Or set the pan over a pilot light on the stove covered with a towel or blanket. The yogurt will take 3 to 5 hours to thicken and then refrigerate. The yogurt can be left to sit overnight and then be refrigerated in the morning. Very good and cheap to make. Try it.

Mexican Style Quinoa

This dish is similar to "Spanish rice" and can be varied by adding other vegetables if desired. When I take it to a carry-in I am always asked for the recipe. Quinoa (keen-wah) is very easy to cook with. You need to rinse it well to get rid of its outer coating. It cooks faster than rice and has all the amino acids of a total protein source such as meat.

1 1/2 tsp. oil or unsalted butter
2 clove minced or pressed garlic
5 shallots or 3/4 cup chopped onion
1 1/2 onion chopped
1-2 jalapeno chile pepper (can use canned) If fresh, blister, steam, peel seed & dice
2 1/4 cups of washed quinoa

1 1/2 Tbs. red pepper flakes
1 1/2 tsp. cumin seeds
1/2 tsp. salt
1/4 tsp. black pepper
1 can Italian plum (roma) tomatoes (drained)
5 cups vegetable stock, tomato juice, or water
1 1/2 cup cooked Anasazi beans or pinto beans

In a 3 quart pan heat the oil or butter, and saute garlic, shallots, onion, chili and quinoa. Add the rest of the seasonings and saute 1 minute. Add the vegetable stock and beans and bring to a boil. Reduce heat, cover and simmer for 20 minutes until the liquid is absorbed. Mix gently and be ready to enjoy a delicious meal. Nice served with a green vegetable, spinach salad and warmed tortillas.

This recipe is an adaptation from *Quinoa, The Supergrain: Ancient Food for Today* by Rebecca Wood.

INDEX